Self-Assessment Colour Review

# Veterinary Parasitology

## Hany M Elsheikha
BVSc, MVS, PhD, FRSPH, FHEA, DipEVPC
School of Veterinary Medicine and Science
University of Nottingham, UK


## Jon S Patterson
DVM, PhD, DipACVP
College of Veterinary Medicine
Michigan State University, USA

T0321418

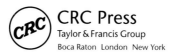

**CRC Press**
Taylor & Francis Group
Boca Raton  London  New York

CRC Press is an imprint of the
Taylor & Francis Group, an **informa** business

# Disclaimer

Therapeutics is an ever-changing field. Readers are advised to check the most up-to-date product information provided by the manufacturer of each drug to verify the recommended dose, the method and duration of administration and adverse effects. It is the responsibility of veterinary practitioners to be familiar with the laws governing drugs in their practice areas and in their country. No responsibility is assumed by the publisher or the authors for any injury and/or damage to persons or property as a matter of products liability, negligence or otherwise, or from any use or operation of any methods, products, instructions or ideas contained in this book. While the use of unlicensed drugs or licensed drugs for unlicensed applications occurs in practice when there are no suitable alternatives, the authors and publisher cannot assume responsibility for the validity of unlicensed drugs mentioned in this book or the consequences of their use. The mention of these drugs is solely for the purpose of specific information and does not imply recommendation or endorsement.

CRC Press
Taylor & Francis Group
6000 Broken Sound Parkway NW, Suite 300
Boca Raton, FL 33487-2742

© 2013 by Taylor & Francis Group, LLC
CRC Press is an imprint of Taylor & Francis Group, an Informa business

ISBN 13: 978-1-84076-188-7 (pbk)

Visit the Taylor & Francis Web site at
http://www.taylorandfrancis.com

and the CRC Press Web site at
http://www.crcpress.com

# Preface

The rationale behind this first edition of *Self-Assessment Colour Review Veterinary Parasitology* developed out of our experience with case-based teaching and teaching parasitology to undergraduate veterinary students for more than 17 years. It became clear as we strived to develop a course that would encourage understanding and enhance learning that parasitology is best taught in a format that fosters students' interest, reasoning and critical thinking. The continuous development and evolution of the discipline of veterinary parasitology add another challenge as concepts change and new discoveries are recognized.

Parasitic diseases are encountered on a daily basis in veterinary practice and there has been a flood of new information in the literature in recent years. This clinically oriented book brings together a wide variety of cases and clinical situations relating to diseases caused by parasitic agents in domestic livestock, wild animals and exotic animals. Each case scenario includes key questions regarding diagnosis, treatment and control of the infection. For example, what are the pearls in the clinical presentation that suggest a specific parasitic agent? How do you interpret these findings? What is the best therapeutic option? The questions are followed by explanatory answers.

This book is not meant to be a reference book, but rather it is a compilation of useful diagnostic scenarios seen in livestock and companion small animals (primarily) and is representative of common parasitic problems. Many of the described situations are accompanied by detailed and challenging epidemiological input, which will encourage the reader to think about differential diagnoses.

There are interesting and important inclusions for exotic species and for fish. Cases are randomly mixed throughout the book, but a broad classification of cases by body system (e.g. cardiovascular, gastrointestinal, nervous) and an index of host and parasite species are provided to guide the reader to specific areas of interest.

With its unique case-based approach, veterinary practitioners, animal health advisers, industry technical representatives, livestock producers and veterinary students should find this book an indispensable addition to the resources they access to expand their knowledge of parasitic diseases of concern and, in addition, be a resource for continuing professional development.

Hany Elsheikha
Jon Patterson

# Contributors

Alexandra Brower, DVM, PhD, DipACVP
School of Veterinary Medicine & Science
University of Nottingham, UK

Peter J Brown, BVS, PhD, DipECVP
School of Veterinary Medicine & Science
University of Nottingham, UK

John E Cooper, DTVM, FRCPath, FSB, CBiol, FRCVS
Department of Veterinary Medicine
University of Cambridge, UK

Hany M Elsheikha, BVSc, MVS, PhD, FRSPH, FHEA, DipEVPC
School of Veterinary Medicine & Science
University of Nottingham, UK

Aiden Foster, BVSc, BSc, PhD, DipACVD, CertSAD, MRCVS
Veterinary Investigation Officer
VLA Shrewsbury, UK

Thomas Geurden, DVM, PhD, DipEVPC
Neesveld 4, 3040 Huldenberg, Belgium

Gayle D Hallowell, MA, VetMB, PhD, CertVA, DipACVIM, MRCVS
School of Veterinary Medicine & Science
University of Nottingham, UK

Craig Hunt, BVetMed, CertSAM, CertZooMed, MRCVS
Chine House Veterinary Hospital
Leicestershire, UK

Steven McOrist, BVSc, PhD, DipECVP
Clinical Associate Professor and Reader
School of Veterinary Medicine & Science
University of Nottingham, UK

Vincent Obanda, BS, MSc
Veterinary Services Department
Kenya Wildlife Service, Nairobi, Kenya

Jon S Patterson, DVM, PhD, DipACVP
Department of Pathobiology & Diagnostic Investigation
Diagnostic Center for Population & Animal Health
College of Veterinary Medicine
Michigan State University, USA

Antonio Ortega Rivas, BPharm, PhD
Faculty of Pharmacy
University Institute of Tropical Diseases & Public Health of the Canary Islands
University of La Laguna, Spain

Paul Sands, BSc, BVetMed, CertVD, MRCVS
Scarsdale Veterinary Group, Derby, UK

Neil Sargison, BA, VetMB, PhD, DSHP, DipECSRHM, FRCVS
Royal (Dick) School of Veterinary Studies
University of Edinburgh, UK

Christina Tellefsen, BVSc, MRCVS
46 Dudley Street
Leighton Buzzard, UK

Chun-Ren Wang, BVSc, MVetSc, PhD
College of Animal Science & Veterinary Medicine
Heilongjiang Bayi Agricultural University
Daqing, People's Republic of China

Paolo Zucca, DVM, PhD
Zooanthropology Unit
Healthcare Services Agency
Trieste, Italy

# Abbreviations

| | | | |
|---|---|---|---|
| ALP | alkaline phosphatase | IFA | indirect fluorescent antibody |
| ALT | alanine aminotransferase | IgG | immunoglobulin G |
| AST | aspartate aminotransferase | IGR | insect growth regulator |
| Bands | immature neutrophils | IH | intermediate hosts |
| BBB | blood–brain barrier | IM | intramuscular |
| BRSV | bovine respiratory syncytial virus | IV | intravenous |
| | | L1 | first-stage larva |
| BUN | blood urea nitrogen | L2 | second-stage larva |
| BVD | bovine viral diarrhoea | L3 | third-stage larva |
| BW | body weight | L4 | fourth-stage larva |
| CBC | complete blood count | MCH | mean corpuscular haemoglobin |
| CK | creatine kinase | | |
| CNS | central nervous system | MCHC | mean corpuscular haemoglobin concentration |
| CPK | creatine phosphokinase | | |
| CSF | cerebrospinal fluid | MCV | mean cell volume |
| CT | computed tomography | MF | microfilariae |
| CVSM | cervical vertebral stenotic myelopathy | ML | macrocyclic lactone |
| | | MRI | magnetic resonance imaging |
| DIC | disseminated intravascular coagulation | NSAID | nonsteroidal anti-inflammatory drug |
| DMSO | dimethyl sulphoxide | PAIR | puncture, aspiration, injection and re-aspiration |
| DNA | deoxyribonucleic acid | | |
| DSH | domestic shorthair | PCR | polymerase chain reaction |
| EDM | equine degenerative myelopathy | PCV | packed cell volume/ haematocrit |
| EEE | Eastern equine encephalitis | PI-3 | parainfluenza-3 (virus) |
| EGS | equine grass sickness | PO | per os |
| EL4 | early fourth stage larvae | PT | post treatment |
| ELISA | enzyme-linked immunosorbent assay | RA | right atrium |
| | | RBCs | red blood cells |
| EM | encysted metacercariae | RLB | reverse line blot hybridization |
| epg | eggs per gram | | |
| EPM | equine protozoal myeloencephalitis | RMSF | Rocky Mountain spotted fever |
| GABA | gamma-aminobutyric acid | RV | right ventricle |
| GGT | gamma glutamyl transferase | SACs | South American camelids |
| GI | gastrointestinal | SC | subcutaneous |
| Hb | haemoglobin | Segmenters | mature neutrophils |
| HCl | hydrochloric acid | TCBZ | triclabendazole |
| H&E | haematoxylin and eosin | WBCs | white blood cells |
| IBR | infectious bovine rhinotracheitis | WNV | West Nile virus |

# Acknowledgements

This book brings together a diverse group of authors from four continents, including experts in a variety of disciplines from academia, industry, research and private practice settings. We are profoundly grateful to all the authors who contributed their time and effort to this book.

All the cases were reviewed by eminent parasitologists from Europe and North America, and we would like to thank them for their detailed comments and helpful suggestions.

The support and encouragement of the staff at Manson Publishing, in particular Jill Northcott, Michael Manson, Paul Bennett and Peter Beynon, has been superb and we are indebted to them all for their help.

Lastly, we would like to express our gratitude to and respect for all of those dedicated colleagues who have committed themselves to the field of veterinary parasitology.

# Image acknowledgements

**5a** Courtesy Mrs Nicole Shultz and Mr Charles Musitano

**150a, b, 190** Courtesy Dr Mike Targett

**42a, b** From Craig M (2011) *Culicoides* hypersensitivity in horses. *UKVET Companion Animal* **16**(4):5–9, with permission

**57** Courtesy IDEXX Laboratories Inc.

**86a, b** From Elsheikha HM (2009) Human health risk implications of ocular myxoboliosis in fish. *Veterinary Times* **39**(9):26–27, with permission.

**100a, b, 103** Courtesy Dr Joe Rook

**112a** Courtesy Dr Mark Stidworthy

**130** Courtesy Dr Michael Scott

**132a, 142** Courtesy Edward Elkan Reference Collection

**141a, b, 154, 166b** Illustration by Mr Richard Cooke

**162, 172** Courtesy Michigan State University, Diagnostic Center for Population and Animal Health

**163a** From Bartley D (2011) Anthelmintic resistance in cattle nematodes Part 1: a problem for the future. *UKVET Livestock* **16**(6):19–22, with permission

**188a–c** From Elsheikha HM, Brown P, Middleton B (2011) Soft thoracic subcutaneous mass in a rabbit (*Oryctolagus cuniculus*). *Lab Animal Europe* **11**(11):10–14, with permission

**189** Courtesy Dr John W McGarry

# Classification of cases by organ systems

Note: Some cases appear under more than one system. Numbers in bold denote cases that have zoonotic implications.

Cardiovascular: 14, 23, 89, 112, **126**, **140**, 159, 164, **176**, 191

Gastrointestinal: 1, 2, 3, 4, 6, 9, 18, 25, 26, 29, 32, **33**, **35**, 41, 43, 45, 47, 54, 55, 57, 60, 62, 63, 67, 72, 80, 81, 85, 91, 100, **101**, 102, 103, 105, 107, **108**, 118, 120, 121, 143, 144, 145, 147, 148, 151, 152, 153, 156, 158, **167**, **169**, 171, 172, 177, 180, 183, 187, **189**, **190**, 193, 194, 195, **197**, 198, 201, 203, 205, **206**, **207**

Liver and pancreas: 1, 26, 61, 63, 69, 87, **110**, **149**, 162, 165, 175, **178**, **190**, 202

Nervous: 12, 13, 16, **33**, 34, 46, 51, 76, 78, 82, 83, 90, 106, 115, 116, 123, **146**, **150**

Ocular: 20, 86

Polysystemic: 21, 71, 91, 97, 104, 119, 125, 130, 132, 136, 141, **170**, 173, 192

Respiratory: 2, 10, 15, 22, 27, 36, 37, 65, 66, 77, **124**, 133, 139, 154, 163, 174, 179, 198, 203

Skin, muscles and soft tissue: 3, 5, 7, 8, 11, 17, 19, 24, **28**, 30, 31, **33**, **38**, **39**, 42, 44, 48, 49, 50, **52**, **53**, 56, 58, 59, 64, 68, 70, 73, **74**, 75, 77, 79, 84, 86, 88, 91, 92, 93, 94, 95, 96, **97**, 98, 99, **106**, 109, 111, 112, 113, 114, 117, 122, **126**, 127, 128, 129, 131, 134, 135, 137, 138, 142, 155, 157, 160, **161**, 166, 168, 181, **182**, 184, 185, 186, 188, **199**, **196**, 200, 204

Urogenital: 40, **146**, **170**

# About the authors

**Hany Elsheikha** is a Lecturer in the Division of Veterinary Medicine at the University of Nottingham School of Veterinary Medicine and Science, UK. He is a board-certified veterinary parasitologist with over 18 years of research and teaching experience in veterinary parasitology. He has authored more than 120 peer-reviewed and lay publications and authored the book titled *Essentials of Veterinary Parasitology*. His research interests include host–parasite interactions and development of novel antiparasitic therapeutics.

**Jon Patterson** is a Professor in the Department of Pathobiology and Diagnostic Investigation and the Diagnostic Center for Population and Animal Health at Michigan State University College of Veterinary Medicine, USA. He is a board-certified veterinary pathologist with over 24 years of experience in teaching, research and diagnostic service. His research interests include student assessment in veterinary education and diseases of the nervous system.

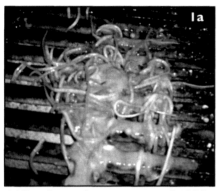
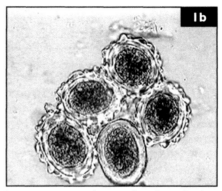

1 The viscera from a group of 100-kg pigs are presented at a slaughter facility with multifocal fibrotic lesions in their livers and noticeable nematodes within the small intestine (1a). The pigs had been raised in a semi-outdoor management farm system with groups of 30- to 100-kg pigs kept on the same site. A faecal flotation examination of cohort 90-kg pigs is made (1b).
i. What is your parasitic diagnosis, and what is the prepatent period of this parasite?
ii. Explain why this problem is less likely on a conventional indoor pig farm.
iii. What treatments are most suitable for this problem?

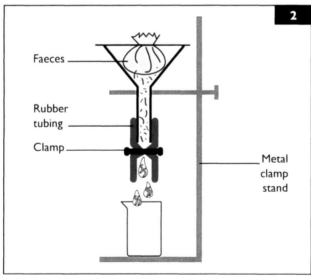

2 What is this apparatus (2)?

## 1, 2: Answers

**1 i.** Intestinal parasitism due to the nematode *Ascaris suum*. Its life cycle includes larval movement through the liver and lungs, then maturity in the intestines, with a 6- to 8-week prepatent period after ingestion of an infective ascarid egg from residual faecal material. Larval movement of *A. suum* is the cause of the 'milk spot' liver lesions.
**ii.** The incidence of ascariosis declined with the construction of indoor farms in the 1970s, with raised, slatted concrete floors breaking the oral–faecal cycle. The incidence is increasing again and is significantly higher in outdoor and 'organic' farm systems. Infection of farm sites requires only a small number of infected pigs from variable sources to enter the site. The thick-coated *A. suum* eggs (**1b**) are highly stable and infectious in the environment of outdoor systems for several years.
**iii.** Endemically infected farms should employ on-going medication programmes. Routine benzimidazoles or ivermectins are adequate. Medication is aimed at prevention of mature intestinal infections by medicating finisher pigs at monthly intervals. In outdoor pig systems, careful attention must be paid to stock management, with field rotations, light stocking densities and regular anthelmintic treatment. Clearing sites of ascarid eggs is not practical unless floor surfaces can be flame treated.

**2** A Baermann apparatus, used to detect, separate and concentrate larvae from faeces, grass, tissue or soil. The Baermann technique is based on active migration or movement of larvae from the faeces, minced tissue, grass or soil into water of a warmer temperature, which is brought into contact with the bottom of the material to be examined. Faeces are suspended in lukewarm water. The larvae move into the water, sink to the bottom and are collected for identification. Larvae may be observed migrating into the water within 10–15 minutes (usually); however, the largest recovery can be obtained by allowing the material to remain in the funnel for 24 hours. The technique is used mainly for diagnosing lungworm infection and for isolating larvae from a faecal culture. It is relatively insensitive for low larvae intensities, therefore sequential samples taken days apart should be obtained and analysed.

3 A 12-year-old Thoroughbred horse is presented in late autumn as an emergency because of signs of distress. On arrival at the livery yard you note that the horse has a bloody tail head (3) from rubbing on the walls of the stable. The whole livery yard has a worming protocol that involves a yearly rotation of dewormers and this year the horses have been dewormed with ivermectin every 8 weeks and were treated for tapeworm infection 2 months ago with an appropriate dose of pyrantel. Physical examination reveals no

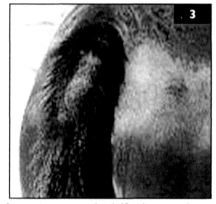

other obvious abnormalities, although the horse is extremely difficult to evaluate because of its stressed condition.
i. What is your differential diagnosis for this case?
ii. How would you confirm your most likely diagnosis?
iii. Why might this animal have this condition despite regular anthelmintic treatment?
iv. How might you treat this animal?

4 A 12-week-old dwarf lop rabbit is presented with a history of acute lethargy and diarrhoea. A fresh faecal smear reveals large numbers of two different organisms (4).
i. Identify the larger organism.
ii. Identify the smaller organisms.
iii. How would you treat this patient?

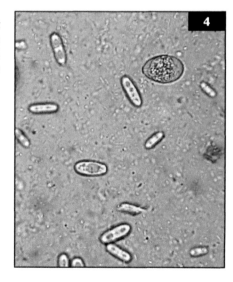

# 3, 4: Answers

**3 i.** The most likely differential diagnosis is *Oxyuris equi* (pinworm) infection. Other possible causes include *Culicoides* hypersensitivity (although not likely at this time of year, and there likely would be some mane involvement), a foreign body embedded within or beneath the tail head and irritation of the perineum (e.g. secondary to loose faeces).
**ii.** Adult pinworms are found in the colon. However, adult female worms migrate to the anus to deposit eggs, which are then cemented in the perianal region. Diagnosis is made by microscopic evaluation of sellotape preparations taken from around the anus.
**iii.** In this horse it seems most likely that either the drug had not been administered or that the horse had received a sub-therapeutic dose. Questioning revealed that the horse was extremely difficult to deworm.
**iv.** A suitable anthelmintic needs to be administered and assessment of the horse's worm burden performed. Options include a different oral anthelmintic (which the clients were unwilling to administer) or, alternatively, administration of a parenteral avermectin administered off-label with warnings of potential adverse consequences. A worm egg count in this animal revealed that there were <50 epg. However, worm egg counts are very insensitive for *Oxyuris* eggs and are not normally used in this situation because the worms produce eggs in the perianal region. Management of the excoriated, oozing wound should include oral prednisolone and topical broad-spectrum antimicrobial ointment. Antimicrobials may be required if the pruritus does not improve quickly.

**4 i.** Coccidia (*Eimeria* species) oocyst; 13 species of intestinal *Eimeria* have been described in the rabbit, the two most pathogenic being *E. magna* and *E. irresidua*. A single species, *E. stiedae*, affects the liver. Oocysts of all species are excreted in the faeces.
**ii.** *Saccharomyces guttulatus*, a commensal yeast.
**iii.** Toltrazuril (25 mg/kg PO for 2 days, repeated after 5 days), trimethoprim/sulphadiazine (30 mg/kg PO q12h for 7 days) or trimethoprim/sulphamethoxazole (40 mg/kg PO q12h for 7 days) are all effective against coccidiosis. *Saccharomyces* requires no treatment.

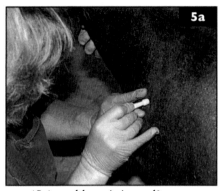

5 What is this instrument (5a), and how is it used?

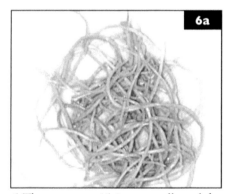
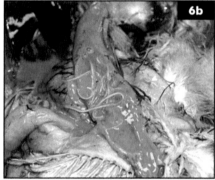

6 These worms (6a) were collected from the small intestine of a chicken during post-mortem examination (6b).
i. What are these worms? How do chickens become infected?
ii. What is their clinical significance?
iii. What treatment and control options would you recommend?

5 A biopsy punch, a surgical instrument used to punch a hole through the uppermost layers of the skin to collect a sample of skin tissue. Skin punch biopsy is a quick, simple and safe procedure and a valuable aid in diagnosing many skin conditions. It offers a suitable histological specimen with a minimum amount of scarring and little or no discomfort to the patient. Some skin biopsies can be done with injection of local anaesthetic (e.g. lidocaine) into the subcutaneous tissue. When using a punch biopsy, rotate in one direction and

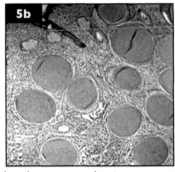

use the punch only once as the blade is easily dulled and may cause the tissue to tear during the procedure. Use the 6- or 7-mm size punches because they provide a good sample size. There are a number of parasitic skin infections for which punch biopsy and histopathology are important tools for confirming the diagnosis. For example, a punch biopsy taken from a donkey with skin lesions that failed to respond to conventional treatments was processed for histopathology with H&E staining. Microscopical examination revealed parasite cysts of *Besnoitia* species in the skin (**5b**), therefore more specific treatment was decided based on these findings.

**6 i.** The ascarid nematode *Ascaridia galli*, a common parasite of chickens. Birds become infected via ingestion of ascarid egg-contaminated food or water. Earthworms may act as paratenic hosts.

**ii.** *A. galli* infection can cause reduced weight gain and feed efficiency, diarrhoea and death, but it is not generally a problem in broiler chickens because of the short grow-out time. These clinical signs are due to toxins produced by the worms, which adversely influence enzyme systems of the intestinal mucosa and interfere with the normal digestion and absorption of nutrients.

**iii.** Most anthelmintics, including fenbendazole, piperazine, levamisole and ivermectin, are effective. Regular deworming every 2–3 months may be necessary. Control also involves breaking the life cycle by reducing contact with the source of contamination (e.g. faeces) by caging. Good sanitation (e.g. removal of dead birds, removal of contaminated litter) followed by disinfection and restrictions on the movement of equipment and personnel can help reduce infection, especially when parasite numbers become excessive. Birds of different ages should not be raised in close proximity, as older birds can serve as a reservoir for infection of young birds.

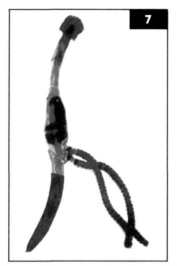

7 This organism (7) was isolated from the gills of a catfish.
i. What is it?
ii. Is it male or female?
iii. What is its clinical significance?
iv. How would you treat infested fish?

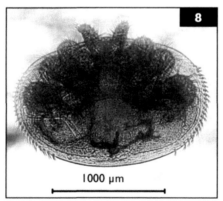

1000 µm

8 This organism (8) was found on a dead European honey bee.
i. What is it?
ii. Is it important?
iii. What is the link between this organism and decreased bee populations?
iv. What recent change has allowed this organism to become more problematic?

**7 i.** The crustacean copepod parasite *Lamproglena* species. Diagnosis of copepod infestation can be made by gross visualization or wet mount examination.
**ii.** An adult female. Mature females are differentiated based on the presence of two easily recognized egg sacs.
**iii.** The impact of *Lamproglena* infestation can range from mild pathological damage to stress-induced mortality of infested fish. Also, during the infestation process the damage and minor wounds caused by attachment and feeding of *Lamproglena* may afford portals of entry to more serious secondary bacterial, viral and fungal infections.
**iv.** There is no ideal treatment. However, organophosphates can be effective; prolonged immersion treatment should be repeated weekly for 4 weeks. Diflubenzuron is less toxic to fish and is effective. It is not inactivated at high temperatures, as are organophosphates. However, diflubenzuron can be harmful to non-target arthropods. Formalin or potassium permanganate baths are also effective. Formalin is carcinogenic and depletes oxygen, so additional aeration is required. Some fish are very sensitive to this treatment. Drugs should be used as part of an integrated health management strategy to mitigate the losses.

**8 i.** *Varroa* mite (*V. destructor* or *V. jacobsoni*).
**ii.** Yes. *Varroa* is a highly damaging ectoparasite of honey bees. The demise of billions of honey bees has been attributed to *Varroa* infestation. The widespread population decline of honey bees on this scale also affects the pollination of economically important crops and exotic plants.
**iii.** *Varroa* feed on the haemolymph of honey bee pupae and adults, and in so doing they transmit infections that reduce the life expectancy of the bees and cause the colony to decline. For example, *Varroa*-borne viral infections can cause permanent physical impairment (e.g. deformed wing virus) or even death of affected bees.
**iv.** Recent climate changes might have allowed increased mite persistence during winter and expansion beyond its normal range, thus increasing the risk of transmission over larger geographical regions.

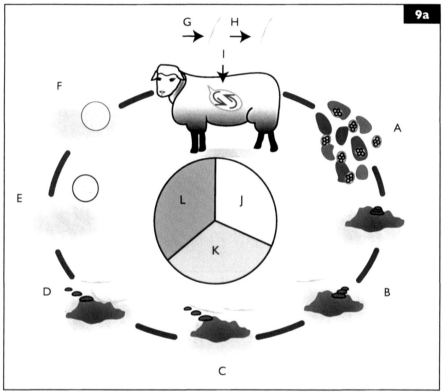

9 i. With which type of parasite is this life cycle (9a) associated?
ii. Name and describe each of the lettered stages.
iii. What are the main clinical signs characterizing acute infection by this parasite?

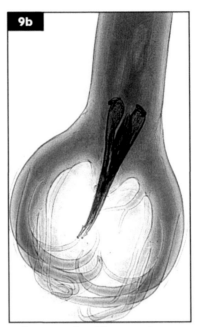

**9 i.** The sheep abomasal nematodes *Haemonchus contortus* and *Teladorsagia circumcincta*. In this case it is *H. contortus* based on the morphology of the male worm posterior end, which has a characteristic bursa (copulatory organ) with its asymmetrical dorsal lobe and y-shaped dorsal ray (**9b**).

**ii.** (A) immature eggs passed in dung; (B) first larval stage (L1) in dung; (C) second larval stage (L2) in dung; (D) third larval stage (L3) in dung; (E) L3 (infective stage) on grass; (F) L3 is eaten in water droplet on grass; (G) L3 moults to fourth larval stage (L4) in abomasal glands; (H) L4 moults to fifth larval stage (L5) in abomasal glands; (I) adult nematode reaches maturity in abomasal lumen; (J) contamination phase; (K) free-living phase; (L) parasitic phase.

**iii.** Anorexia, depression, loss of condition, anaemia and pale mucous membranes due to blood loss. Also, submandibular oedema (bottle jaw) due to the accumulation of fluid caused by hypoproteinaemia.

10 A gamebird farm suffers reduced egg production and increased mortality among the breeding stock. Birds of different species show sneezing, coughing, head shaking and respiratory distress. Some birds open their beaks and stretch their necks, gasping for air ('gaping posture'). Faecal examination reveals a large number of worm eggs (10a).

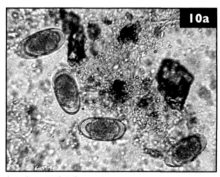

i. What is the name of the parasite that produces these eggs? What anatomical structure(s) is/are primarily affected in birds? Which avian groups are most susceptible to this infection?
ii. What is your differential diagnosis?
iii. What is the suggested treatment?

11 Microscopical examination of a skin scraping from a koi carp during a routine health check reveals this organism (11).
i. What is this organism?
ii. Is it significant?
iii. Describe its life cycle.
iv. What treatment would you advise?

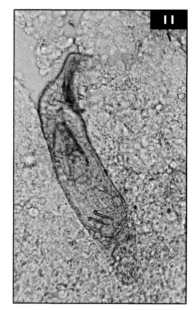

**10 i.** *Syngamus trachea* (**10b**), a 'gapeworm' commonly found in the trachea of gamebirds and pheasants, although it can infect any species of cage and aviary bird. The infection rate in some groups of wild birds is high and young birds are most commonly affected. Fertilized eggs are swallowed by the bird and spread with the faeces or directly expelled onto the ground from the trachea. Earthworms can act as a transport host.

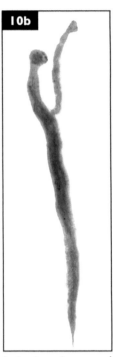

**ii.** Even though the gaping posture is pathognomonic, the differential diagnosis should take into account other conditions that cause respiratory distress (e.g. aspergillosis, mycoplasmosis, tracheal mite infection).

**iii.** It is difficult to control tracheal worm infection in birds kept on the ground in open-air enclosures/aviaries. Therefore, parasitological examination of the faeces should be performed regularly throughout the year. Benzimidazoles are the first-choice drugs and these are usually administered in the feed. (Refer to an avian/exotic animal formulary for dosage and duration of treatment.)

**11 i.** *Gyrodactylus* species, a monogenean parasite (skin fluke) of aquatic animals.

**ii.** *Gyrodactylus* flukes feed on the skin and mucus, causing irritation. Stress and injury, as a result of fish attempting to dislodge parasites by rubbing their bodies against substrate and furnishings, predispose to secondary bacterial and fungal infection.

**iii.** *Gyrodactylus* is viviparous/larviparous and has a direct life cycle with the potential to reach high numbers rapidly under favourable conditions.

**iv.** Over-the-counter remedies containing formalin and methylene blue may be successful. Other treatments include sodium chloride (1–5 g/l permanent bath, or 30–35 g/l 4–5 minute bath); mebendazole (1 mg/kg as a 24-hour bath); praziquantel (2–10 mg/l bath for up to 4 hours every 5 days for 3 treatments, or 5–12 g/kg feed q24h for 3 days). Deficiencies in water quality, husbandry and stocking density should be rectified.

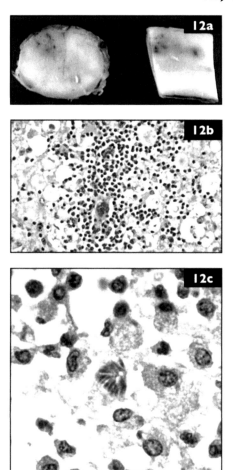

12 A 2.5-year-old Standardbred stallion is euthanized after a 2-month history of progressively worsening ataxia and weakness of all four limbs, with severity one grade worse in the hindlimbs compared with the forelimbs. There is also moderate gluteal muscle atrophy on the right side and the tail is hypotonic. The horse's appetite has decreased steadily over the past 2 weeks. The tentative clinical diagnosis is EPM. Examination of formalin-fixed spinal cord reveals grey-brown discolouration of the ventral grey and white matter in the C2 and L6 spinal cord segments (12a). Histopathological sections were obtained (12b, c). Describe the nature of the inflammatory reaction in the spinal cord if the diagnosis in this case is indeed EPM.

13 What is 'gid'?

12 Granulomatous inflammation, with a predominance of macrophages and lesser numbers of lymphocytes and plasma cells (**12b**). Eosinophils are occasionally seen in cases of EPM. Protozoal organisms (schizonts) are rarely found in chronic lesions, but may be identified more easily in acute lesions (**12c**).

13 Coenurosis ('gid', 'sturdy') is a disease of the brain and spinal cord caused by invasion and development of *Coenurus cerebralis*, the larval stage of *Taenia multiceps*. The disease occurs in sheep and, rarely, in cattle. *C. cerebralis* causes cortical meningitis and encephalitis. Affected sheep hold their head to one side and in some cases the animal turns in circles. There may be unilateral partial blindness, pain response on pressure over the cystic area, paralysis of limbs and pressure atrophy of the brain and bones of the skull adjacent to the cyst. Dogs and other carnivores act as definitive hosts by harbouring adult tapeworms, thus serving as a continuous source of infection through discharge of eggs in the faeces. Eggs excreted from infected dogs contain hexacanth larvae. Sheep become infected via ingestion of eggs with contaminated food or water. Embryos hatch, burrow through the intestinal wall and travel to the brain and spinal cord via the blood. Once in the brain, a cyst develops within several months and grows to a size that results in the onset of clinical signs. When dogs or other canids ingest infected sheep tissue, the parasite develops into the adult tapeworm and passes mature egg-containing segments in the faeces. Fallen carcasses or slaughterhouse-disposed viscera containing mature *Coenurus* cysts pose a serious threat to dogs or other wild carnivores. Treatment ranges from administering albendazole, niclosamide or praziquantel to surgical removal if the cyst can be located. Controlling coenurosis through vaccination is still at an early stage. The frequency of coenurosis in humans is unknown, but this is a serious zoonosis and can lead to pathological conditions in affected humans.

**14** A 4-year-old neutered male DSH cat was found dead. At necropsy, the heart's appearance was consistent with hypertrophic cardiomyopathy (HCM). Histopathological assessment revealed large numbers of cystic structures (**14**) in sections of skeletal muscles (neck, intercostal muscles and diaphragm) and in cardiac muscle.

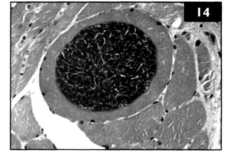

**i.** What is the most likely diagnosis?
**ii.** How would you confirm the diagnosis?
**iii.** How did the cat get these cysts?
**iv.** What is the link between cardiomyopathy and these cysts?

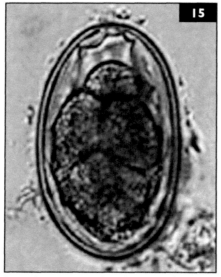

**15** A 3-year-old female owl is presented with severe dyspnoea and very poor body condition. A swab of the oropharynx reveals large numbers of inflammatory cells, but no aetiological agents. Several nematode eggs, each with a barely visible operculum and 8 blastomeres (**15**), are seen on faecal examination.
**i.** What is your diagnosis?
**ii.** How would you treat this owl?

**14 i.** The cysts have morphological features consistent with sarcocysts of *Sarcocystis* species, most likely *S. felis*. Usually, cats infected with *S. felis* sarcocysts are asymptomatic and a diagnosis is made if the cat has a concomitant infection or condition, as in this case.

**ii.** A tentative diagnosis is based on clinical history, post-mortem and histopathological examinations and serological tests (e.g. IFA for IgG antibodies against *S. cruzi*, *S. neurona* or *Toxoplasma gondii*). Confirmation is by DNA sequencing and phylogenetic analyses. Electron microscopy will reveal ultrastructural features of the bradyzoites and wall of the sarcocystis cysts.

**iii.** *Sarcocystis* species have a two-host life cycle. Cats act as the definitive host by harbouring *Sarcocystis* oocysts in their intestines. They can also serve as an IH by developing sarcocysts in their muscles. Sarcocysts have been reported in skeletal and cardiac muscles of cats, where the animals were severely compromised by diseases other than sarcocystosis (e.g. pancytopenia, metastatic neoplasia, generalized lymphosarcoma, HCM). It is difficult to determine whether the cysts in this cat were derived from oocysts/sporocysts through faecal–oral autoinfection or from other carnivores. Immunosuppression has been suggested as a reason for the unusual presence of sarcocysts in cats, as indicated above. This cat was in good condition and showed no evidence of an impaired immune system.

**iv.** The low prevalence of sarcocysts in cardiac muscles suggests that an association between the parasite cysts and HCM is probably coincidental. HCM is a common cause of sudden death in cats and usually results in hypertrophy and stiffness of cardiac muscles. HCM mostly occurs in middle-aged animals; however, it has been reported in kittens as young as 2 months old. The condition may be due to an autosomal recessive mode of inheritance or other genetic components. The aetiology in this case remains unknown.

**15 i.** *Syngamus (Cyathostoma) bronchialis*. *Syngamus trachea* is also a possibility.
**ii.** With benzimidazoles or levamisole via the water. One week post treatment a faecal check revealed no eggs, but the owl died within 10 days following treatment.

**16** You are presented with a 3-year-old Percheron brood mare that is currently 4 months in foal and is housed in a remote area of central California (USA). The mare is asymmetrically ataxic with the left hindlimb worse than the right. You suspect EPM in this case. However, immunofluorescent testing of serum and CSF is positive for *Neospora hughesi*, but negative for *S. neurona*.

**i.** How does the life cycle of *N. hughesi* differ from that of *S. neurona*?

**ii.** What other differences are there between these two organisms?

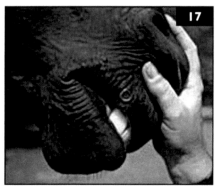

**17** You are asked in late spring to examine a 10-year-old Warmblood gelding that has ulcerated, raised lesions around the corners of its mouth (**17**). The owner reports that these are interfering with the bit. She reports that the horse appears slightly sensitive around the lesions. The horse has no other abnormalities, is regularly dewormed and is vaccinated against influenza and tetanus. For the previous 5 years the horse has shown no evidence of skin disease.

**i.** What is the differential diagnosis for these clinical signs?

**ii.** What is the life cycle of the parasite that is causing these clinical signs?

**iii.** How would you treat and manage this condition?

**16 i.** Less is known about the life cycle of *N. hughesi*. The definitive host for *Neospora caninum* is the domestic dog and this may or may not be the same for *N. hughesi*. Both tachyzoites and tissue cysts have been found in horses.
**ii.** In the USA the seroprevalence of *N. hughesi* is low compared with *S. neurona*, therefore at the present time its role in causing disease is likely to be limited. It has been also identified in Canada and New Zealand. Another key difference is that congenital infections with *N. hughesi* have been confirmed, therefore transplacental transmission occurs, as is found with *N. caninum* in cattle, but not with *S. neurona* in horses. Further research is needed regarding how this protozoan organism causes neurological disease in horses and why the prevalence is so low.

**17 i.** The main differential is cutaneous habronemosis. Other potential differentials include bacterial and fungal granulomas, exuberant granulation secondary to a previous wound or trauma (likely in this case from the bit), squamous cell carcinoma and, potentially, a sarcoid.
**ii.** Adult worms (*Habronema microstoma* and *H. megastoma*) live in the stomach of the horse. Larvae are excreted in the faeces and ingested by house flies (*Musca domestica*) or stable flies (*Stomoxys calcitrans*) in which they mature and become infective. Infective larvae are deposited near the mouth of the horse and swallowed. Lesions on the skin are caused by an inflammatory response to the infective larvae as they are deposited on skin and wounds, which are often wet, as they attempt to migrate to the mouth.
**iii.** By treating the inflammatory response and eliminating the parasite. The former involves the use of oral steroids (prednisolone or dexamethasone); the latter the use of oral ivermectin or moxidectin, which may require a second dose 2–4 weeks later. Fly control is required; topical repellents containing permethrin are the most effective. Proper management of manure is essential to reduce the fly burden around the stables.

18 You are presented with a 12-year-old Thoroughbred-cross mare that has a 4-month history of chronic intermittent colic, with the horse showing signs of abdominal pain approximately once weekly. Each of these episodes responds favourably to the administration of intravenous phenylbutazone. Transabdominal ultrasonography reveals no abnormalities; the intestinal walls show normal thickness and motility is normal. Biopsy of the pyloric antrum reveals granulomatous tissue with a large number of eosinophils and focal areas of necrosis.
i. What is the most likely diagnosis in this case, and what other differential diagnoses would you consider?
ii. Why is this horse showing clinical signs of abdominal pain?
iii. How would you treat this horse?

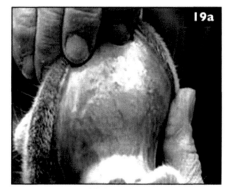 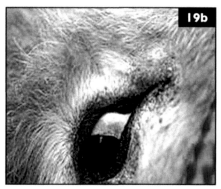

19 A 3-year-old female miniature donkey is presented with multifocal white to yellow pinpoint glistening papules (up to 1 mm in diameter) in the submucosa of the inner lip (19a), ocular sclera (19b), eyelids and external nares.
i. What is your diagnosis?
ii. What other clinical signs would be present in this condition?
iii. How would you confirm the diagnosis?
iv. What are the therapeutic options for managing this case?

# 18, 19: Answers

**18 i.** Gastric habronemosis. Possible differential diagnoses include gastric squamous cell carcinoma, exuberant response to *Gasterophilus* species larvae and severe gastric ulceration.

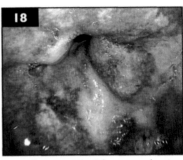

**ii.** Because there is an intermittent obstruction of the pylorus (18). When the stomach fills and cannot empty, stretch receptors will be activated.

**iii.** Oral ivermectin or moxidectin is effective, although one or more doses may be required at 2-week intervals. Fly control using topical repellents and good management of manure is required to reduce the fly burden around the stables.

**19 i.** Besnoitiosis, an infectious disease of equids caused by the intracellular protozoan *Besnoitia bennetti*.

**ii.** Focal areas of rough lichenified skin with raised small dermal nodules on the head, the base of the ears, the shoulders and the inner aspects of the hindlimbs as well as the perineal and perivulvar regions. Multifocal to coalescing areas of alopecia and hypotrichosis, with thickened, irregular, crusty, hyperpigmented skin, can be found on the neck, around the muzzle and eyes and on the distal extremities. The severity of the lesions can vary from mild thickening with slight superficial scaling to marked thickening associated with hyperpigmentation, fissuring and epidermal ulceration with serous exudation and crust formation.

**iii.** Histological examination of skin biopsies of affected lesions and demonstration of thick-walled *Besnoitia* cysts, 0.1–0.5 mm diameter (see **6b**), within infected skin and ocular lesions.

**iv.** There is no effective treatment because most infections are followed by cyst formation, with a thick cyst wall, that is impermeable to therapeutic agents. Trimethoprim and sulphamethoxazole may have some prophylactic and therapeutic value if given early in the course of disease. Daily treatment of donkeys with trimethoprim (1.0 mg/kg) and sulphamethoxazole (20 mg/kg) for 42 days can lead to some clinical improvement. Donkeys treated with trimethoprim (160 mg) and sulphamethoxazole (800 mg) tablets (5 tablets daily) for 7 months showed clinical improvement. Pruritic dermatitis resolved in a donkey medicated with sulphamethoxazole for 30 days, discontinued for 30 days and then treated for an additional 30 days, but results have not been validated by biopsy.

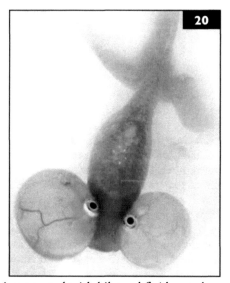

20 A fancy goldfish is presented with bilateral fluid cysts beneath the eyes (20).
i. What is the cause of these structures?
ii. How would you treat the condition?

21 How might an ELISA be useful in the diagnosis of parasitic disease?

**20 i.** This is a 'normal' fancy variety of goldfish called a 'bubble eye'.
**ii.** No treatment is required.

**21** An ELISA is a serological test used for immunodiagnosis of parasitic infections. It can be used for testing for humoral immune responses (i.e. antibody titres) against parasites (**21A**) or for the presence of parasite antigen (**21B**). In the former, purified parasite antigens are precoated onto an ELISA plate. The patient's serum, which contains antibodies, is incubated on the plate so antibodies react with the fixed antigens. Animal species-specific secondary immunoglobulin coupled with an enzyme is then applied. The enzymes used most often are horseradish peroxidase and alkaline phosphatase, both of which release a dye (chromogen) when exposed to their substrate. The substrate for the enzyme changes colour when cleaved by the enzyme attached to the secondary antibody. Colour development indicates that all the components reacted and that antibody was present in the patient's serum. For the antigen test, the ELISA plate is coated with parasite-specific antibodies and the unknown antigen is bound. The test is read following a second addition of antibody specific to the antigen, which is also conjugated to an enzyme. Lack of colour indicates that the antigen is absent. ELISA is a sensitive, easily run, quantitative test that can be used to determine the presence and level of antibody in the tested serum. However, it is important to consider whether the patient has had time to develop an immune response to a parasite. Monitoring immune responses with ELISA or other serological tests could have a considerable impact on the diagnosis and treatment of parasitic disease and evaluation of therapeutic immune responses. Because false positives occur, a verification test may be necessary (e.g. Western blot).

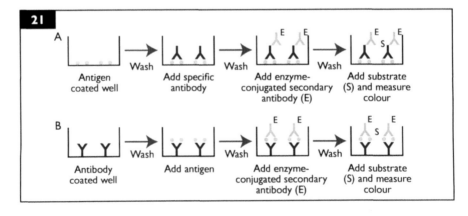

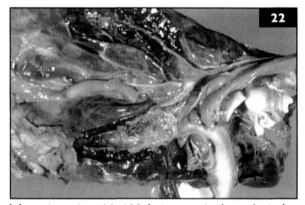

**22** Groups of fattening pigs (30–120 kg) are raised partly indoors and partly outdoors with access to apples and other fallen fruits in a large open orchard. Some of the older pigs develop poor body condition and a deep hacking cough. A faecal flotation from affected pigs shows occasional small embryonated eggs. At post-mortem examination of one affected pig, numerous worms are found in the bronchial tree (**22**).
**i.** What are these worms?
**ii.** Describe this parasite's life cycle.
**iii.** How do these worms cause damage in the lungs of the pig?

**23 i.** As a clinician, how would you describe 'vena caval syndrome', caused by the parasite *Dirofilaria immitis*, to a client?
**ii.** How would you treat a dog with vena caval syndrome?

# 22, 23: Answers

**22 i.** The pig lungworm *Metastrongylus apri*, a slender nematode worm, up to 50 mm in length, found in the small bronchi and bronchioles of the lungs.
**ii.** The life cycle is indirect. Eggs are laid by adult worms in the bronchi and then coughed up, swallowed and passed out via the faeces. They are eaten by earthworms in which they develop through larval stages over 10 days to become infective. The cycle is completed by the pig eating the infected earthworm. Infection, therefore, only occurs where pigs have access to earthworms (e.g. outdoor farms with open ground). Ingested larvae within the earthworms penetrate the intestinal wall and migrate via the lymph nodes and blood vessels to the lungs. The prepatent period is 3–4 weeks.
**iii.** The damage is primarily due to irritation as the larvae migrate through the lungs, and the presence of the worms and their eggs in the bronchi. This produces a persistent cough and mild pneumonia. The lung damage can precipitate or enhance other respiratory diseases. Growth rates may be impaired. Control is by preventing access to infected earthworms.

**23 i.** Caval syndrome is a severe complication of heartworm disease in dogs associated with the presence of a large number of worms in the right ventricle (RV), the right atrium (RA) and the vena cava (VC). Tangled masses of worms in the VC and RA (**23**) interfere with blood return and disrupt the tricuspid valve apparatus, causing tricuspid regurgitation. The syndrome is characterized by acute onset of anorexia, lethargy, weakness, respiratory distress and dark red urine. Clinical signs result from cardiogenic shock, intravascular haemolysis and right heart failure.
**ii.** (1) administration of oxygen to relieve the hypoxaemia caused by poor cardiac output; (2) intravenous fluid administration to support circulation; (3) blood transfusion to stabilize the patient prior to worm removal; (4) anti-inflammatory doses of glucocorticosteroids and heparin prior to worm removal because of the risks of antigen release and anaphylactic reaction (associated with worm maceration) and thromboembolism; and (5) surgical worm removal via jugular venotomy with the use of a long (20–40 cm), small diameter, flexible alligator forceps, preferably using echocardiographic or fluoroscopic guidance. Owners should be advised that prognosis is guarded to poor, with a mortality rate of 30–40%, and that strict rest must be enforced.

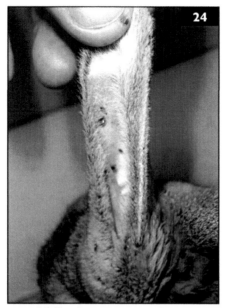

24 A pet rabbit is presented following recapture after straying among a wild rabbit population. Several organisms (24) are identified firmly attached to the pinnae.
i. What are these organisms?
ii. What is their significance?
iii. How would you treat this condition? What treatment should you avoid and why?

25 A captive bird of prey presents with clinical signs of regurgitation. A biopsy of the bird's crop reveals parasites (25).
i. What are these parasites?
ii. What is their clinical significance, and how are they transmitted?
iii. How might this infection be treated or controlled?

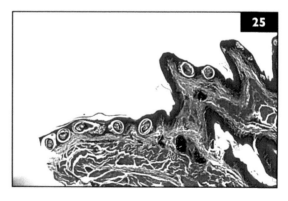

**24 i.** Rabbit fleas, *Spilopsyllus cuniculi*, easily recognized by their predilection for the pinnae. Rabbits may also be infested with cat and dog fleas (*Ctenocephalides felis* and *C. canis*, respectively), though these have a predilection for the dorsum and tail base. Species identity is confirmed by looking at the arrangement of the genal and pronotal combs (spines).
**ii.** Fleas can cause severe pruritus and cutaneous hypersensitivity reactions and in severe infestations may cause anaemia. Rabbit fleas are an important vector in two fatal viral infections of rabbits: myxomatosis and viral haemorrhagic disease.
**iii.** Imidacloprid is the only licensed treatment for rabbit fleas in the UK. Selamectin (6–18 mg/kg) appears effective and safe. Fipronil, while effective against fleas, has caused fatal reactions in rabbits and is therefore not recommended. Flea collars should be avoided. Not only can rabbits hurt themselves trying to bite the collar off, the chemical dosage on the flea collar is generally at toxic levels. Flea dips and powders should also be avoided. Baths are stressful for rabbits, as they can go into shock. It is important to treat the environment because this is where the eggs and larvae live and develop. Treatment of all in-contact animals is advisable. A spot-on solution should be applied to the back of the rabbit's neck where the rabbit cannot lick it off. Segregate treated rabbits so they cannot lick the medication off each other's backs; ingestion of topical medications can cause stomach problems.

**25 i.** Nematodes, formerly called *Capillaria contorta*, now renamed *Eucoleus contortus*.
**ii.** As the history indicates, these worms can be one cause of regurgitation in birds of prey – so-called 'oesophageal capillariosis'. Other causes of such clinical signs include bacterial infections, candidosis and trichomonosis. The life cycle is direct. Transmission is usually from one bird to another following ingestion of eggs.
**iii.** Worms can be killed using anthelmintics (e.g. ivermectin, fenbendazole or mebendazole). Control measures involve good hygiene to reduce the spread of parasites from bird to bird.

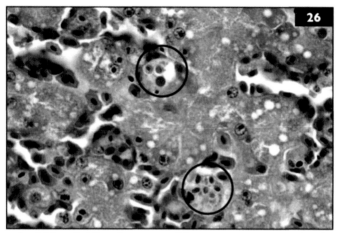

26 A 9-month-old female Rhea is presented for post-mortem examination. There is a significant amount of mucus in the oropharynx and a small amount in the caudal portion of the oesophagus. On histopathological examination, the caeca show severe, subacute, diffuse, fibrinous and necrotizing typhlitis with pale staining, 5–20 micron bodies. The liver also has numerous similar bodies (circled) within sinusoids (26).

i. What is the likely aetiology of these lesions?
ii. How does the bird become infected with this parasite?
iii. How can the disease be managed?

# 26: Answer

**26 i.** The intestinal and hepatic lesions are typical of histomonosis (syns. infectious enterohepatitis or blackhead disease), a disease of gallinaceous birds caused by the protozoan *Histomonas meleagridis*.

**ii.** The protozoan can be transmitted through vectors (caecal worms [*Heterakis gallinarum*] as an IH or earthworms as a paratenic host). Also, the disease can be transmitted horizontally by ingestion of fresh faeces containing live trophozoites. Most blackhead transmission is due to ingesting infected caecal worm eggs. Direct transmission of *H. meleagridis* by 'cloacal drinking' may occur whenever the cloaca of the bird comes into contact with infected fresh droppings. Histomonads may then be transferred into the cloaca by the cloacal reflex and into the caeca by reverse peristalsis. After initial infection, the flagellated histomonad resides in the caeca before invading the intestinal tissue. The histomonad undergoes a flagellate-to-amoeba transformation during tissue invasion and then travels to the liver through the portal vein, causing necrotic liver lesions.

**ii.** Good management is the most effective method of preventing histomonosis as many of the effective drugs used in past years are no longer available commercially. Caecal worm control is necessary to reduce the incidence of blackhead disease. Drugs that reduce the presence of caecal worms, and thus reduce the infection rate, are available but do not have any effect on *Histomonas* organisms. Because healthy chickens often carry infected caecal worms, any contact between chickens and Rhea should be avoided. Grouse and quail also may carry infection to Rhea yards. Because *H. gallinarum* eggs can survive in soil for many months or years, Rhea should not be put on ground contaminated by chickens or turkeys.

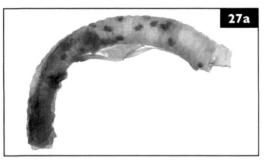

27 During a post-mortem examination, several tiny mites are found inside the trachea of a canary (27a).
i. What is this parasite?
ii. Which avian species are mostly affected?
iii. What are the main clinical signs of infection? What is the differential diagnosis?
iv. What treatment should be used?

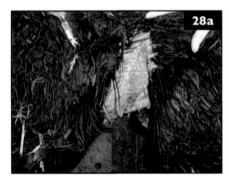

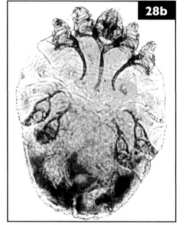

28 A 4-year-old female llama is presented with poor body condition, pruritus, thickened skin, alopecia, erythema and crust formation, mainly distributed over the ventral abdomen (28a). The face and ears are also affected. Scrapings are taken from skin of the affected areas (28b).
i. What is this organism, and is it significant?
ii. Describe the histopathological features associated with this condition.
iii. How can this problem be treated and prevented?

# 27, 28: Answers

27 i. *Sternostoma tracheacolum*, a lung mite that is distributed worldwide (27b).

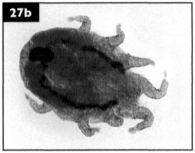

ii. Sternostomosis has been recorded in canaries and in several other species of captive and wild Passeriformes including finches, starlings, blackbirds, orioles, swallows, parrots, parakeets and sparrows.

iii. Clinical signs are related to respiratory distress (open mouth breathing, coughing, sneezing, tail bobbing). These signs are not pathognomonic because bacterial (e.g. *Mycoplasma*) and viral (e.g. avian pox) infections can cause similar signs. Isolation of the mite from the trachea, lungs or other portions of the respiratory tract is required for a definitive diagnosis.

iv. Ivermectin suspension as a spot-on or pyrethroid (or derivates such as permethrin) delivered via aerosol. (Refer to an avian formulary tailored to medicines available in individual countries for appropriate dosages, timings and duration of therapy.)

28 i. *Sarcoptes scabiei* var. *auchinae*, the causative agent of sarcoptic mange. Sarcoptic mange is a potentially serious clinical problem in llamas and other South American camelids. The mite is very contagious and has the ability to cause serious clinical disease on a herd level, especially when inappropriate treatments are administered.

ii. Histopathological examination of affected skin may show multifocal hyperkeratosis, parakeratosis, acanthosis, a large number of mites within the epidermis, multifocal to coalescent crust formation, multifocal superficial infiltration and epidermal transmigration of a mixed inflammatory cell population including eosinophils, multifocal to coalescent pigmentary incontinence, absence of hair follicles and occasional microabscesses. The pathogenic effects of these mites have been attributed to their burrowing activity and the mechanical damage caused by the mites during excavation, the irritant action of the mites' secretion and excretion, allergic reactions to some of their extracellular products and the secretion of host inflammatory cytokines.

iii. Subcutaneous injection of ivermectin (0.2 mg/kg body weight every 14 days) should give satisfactory results. Owners need to be educated about the biosecurity risk associated with the introduction of new animals to a herd and the responsible use of drugs that are available without veterinary prescription. The owner should be advised to wear protective clothing when handling this animal because of the zoonotic risk.

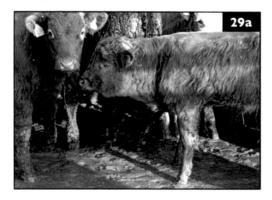

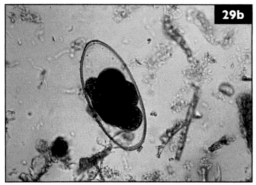

29 At the beginning of December (northern hemisphere), an outbreak of ill thrift with brown, watery diarrhoea and submandibular oedema is investigated in a group of 50 7-month-old weaned beef calves (29a). The cause of the problem is found to be multifactorial, involving fasciolosis, cooperiosis and nematodirosis. The calves had all been treated with a doramectin pour-on anthelmintic drug on arrival at the farm 6 weeks previously. They had then been turned out onto fields that had been grazed by yearling cattle the previous summer. These older cattle had been injected with a depot formulation of moxidectin at turnout in May. Using the McMaster technique, the mean faecal *Nematodirus helvetianus* egg count (29b) of 12 of the 7-month-old calves at the beginning of December is found to be 77 epg, with individual counts ranging from 0 to 550 epg.

i. Are these faecal *N. helvetianus* egg counts significant?

ii. How can the diagnosis of nematodirosis be explained, given the grazing management and anthelmintic treatment history?

# 29: Answer

**29 i.** Yes. A mean count of 77 epg in low dry matter, diarrhoeic faeces represents a very high female worm burden that could be clinically significant; a similar count in high dry matter faeces may be less important.

**ii.** The expectation was that the pastures that had been stocked by yearling cattle, which had been injected with a depot formulation of moxidectin at turnout, would be 'safe'. However, while this treatment will afford 120 days protection against reinfection with *Ostertagia ostertagi*, it will achieve little or no persistence against *N. helvetianus*. It is therefore possible that the absence of *O. ostertagi* from the abomasum of the yearling cattle created an environment that favoured the establishment of *N. helvetianus* and subsequent pasture contamination with *N. helvetianus* eggs. Development to *N. helvetianus* L3s takes place within the egg shell. The critical requirements for hatching of *N. helvetianus* are poorly understood and may differ between populations, as in the case of *N. battus*. The grazing management and anthelmintic treatment history in this case suggests that the *N. helvetianus* eggs did not require a period of chilling before hatching and that pasture L3s could have arisen from egg contamination by the yearling cattle during the same grazing season. However, the possibility of autumn to autumn transmission, requiring overwinter chilling and a high critical hatching temperature, cannot be discounted. In fact, it seems likely that the parasite has the potential to change under the selective pressure of grazing management systems and anthelmintic drug use. It is unlikely that the newly weaned calves would have harboured significant *N. helvetianus* burdens when they arrived on the farm. While pour-on doramectin treatment might have been expected to kill and protect against reinfection with *O. ostertagi* for about 35 days, it would have lacked efficacy against. *N. helvetianus*. Thus, in the absence of a significant modulatory effect of *O. ostertagi*, *N. helvetianus* L3s acquired from contaminated pasture could have given rise to the pathogenic worm burdens seen.

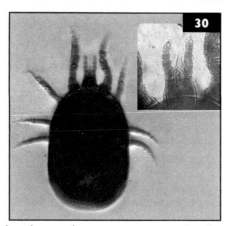

30 Restlessness, reduced growth rate among growing hens and reduced egg production among layers are reported at an egg production facility. Clinical examination reveals skin irritation (manifest as redness), increased feather picking and weight loss. On post-mortem examination, a few tiny dead mites (30) are found on the carcasses.
i. What is the most likely diagnosis?
ii. What treatment and control measures could be recommended?
iii. What are the consequences of this infection?
iv. Are there any zoonotic risks?

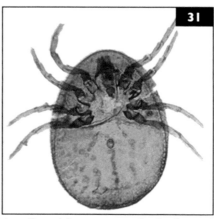

31 This parasite (31) is collected from among the feathers of a laying hen.
i. What is it, and what is its significance?
ii. How can infestation by this parasite be controlled?

**30 i.** Infestation with red mite (*Dermanyssus gallinae*), one of the most serious parasitic diseases of poultry farms in Europe. The mite is a temporary, obligatory haematophagus ectoparasite and spends most of its life cycle hidden in crevices and cracks in the poultry house. It is found on the host only when feeding, usually during the night.

**ii.** Controlling red mite infestation is difficult for several reasons: the life cycle of the mite is very short; it is able to hide itself in small spaces all over the farm; and several antiparasitic drug resistances have been reported. Currently, pyrethroids are the first-choice acaricide drugs used in poultry and non-food birds because of their low toxicity and egg contamination risk. Whenever resistance is suspected, rotation to a different acaricide drug or searching for alternatives to synthetic chemical agents is suggested. The acaricidal effects of plant-derived essential oils (e.g. neem oil) have been tested for red mite control and found to reduce significantly the mite numbers in poultry houses fitted with traps containing 20% oil in water, as compared to those houses that contained traps with water alone. Also, garlic-based acaricides developed for use against poultry red mite appear to hold promise for poultry mite management.

**iii.** Severe from an economical and medical viewpoint. Feeding mites cause irritation, restlessness, anaemia, significant decrease in egg production and increased mortality rates. They may act as a vector for a number of poultry bacterial and viral infections. Therefore, the presence of red mites on the farm should be monitored regularly.

**iv.** Several cases of human infection have been reported, with skin irritation, dermatitis and hypersensitivity to the mite bite, especially in poultry house workers.


**31 i.** *Argas persicus*, a soft tick found in tropical and subtropical areas of the world. It acts as the vector of *Borrelia anserina* (avian spirochetosis) and *Aegyptianella pullorum* (aegyptianellosis). Besides being vectors of some poultry diseases, infestation by this tick can also cause weight loss, depression, decrease in egg production, toxaemia and paralysis. Red spots can be seen on the skin where the ticks have fed. All life cycle stages (larva, nymph and adult) feed several times per night. Because this tick is nocturnal, infested birds may show some uneasiness when roosting. This and other *Argas* species can cause great irritation when feeding on humans.

**ii.** After houses are cleaned, walls, ceilings, cracks and crevices should be treated thoroughly (using a high-pressure sprayer) with carbaryl, coumaphos, malathion, stirofos or a mixture of stirofos and dichlorvos. Cracks and crevices should be filled in.

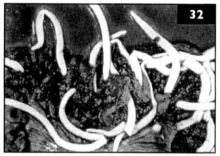

32 Individuals among groups of outdoor farm pigs show mild diarrhoea and poor body condition. The pigs were born and raised outdoors in open-range conditions, with minimal supplementary feeding. At post-mortem examination of one older pig, among other pathological findings there were numerous nodules and long parasites in the small intestine (32).
i. What is the genus and species name of this parasite? To what phylum of parasites does it belong?
ii. Describe these adult worms and their location. Are they pathogenic? On what do they feed?
iii. Describe the unusual life cycle of this parasite.

33 True or false?
i. The presence of fresh blood in the faeces may indicate the presence of a hook-worm infection.
ii. *Notoedres cati* is called the 'walking dandruff' mite of cats.
iii. *Culicoides* hypersensitivity typically lessens in severity with age.
iv. Macrocyclic lactones (MLs) cause starvation and paralysis in treated worms because these compounds open cationic channels, leading to depolarization of nematode muscle cell membrane.
v. It is recommended to treat dogs with whipworm infections monthly for 3 months, as opposed to 2 weeks after an initial treatment, as with most other intestinal worm infections.
vi. Lufenuron is effective against both larvae and adult fleas.

# 32, 33: Answers

**32 i.** *Macracanthorhynchus hirudinaceus* (giant thorny-headed worm). This is an acanthocephalan worm, a rare group, not related to cestodes.

**ii.** They measure 100–400 mm in length and are found within the lumen of the small intestine. The anterior end has a retractile proboscis with six rows of curved hooks, which hold the worm to the small intestinal wall. Large numbers of adult worms can cause considerable damage to the wall of the small intestine due to granulomatous nodule formation. *M. hirudinaceus* lacks any trace of a gut. Feeding is by assimilating nutrients from the intestinal contents of the host.

**iii.** There are male and female adult *M. hirudinaceus* worms, which copulate to fertilize the females' eggs. Females then lay numerous embryonated eggs, which are deposited into nearby soil via the faeces of host pigs. The white larval grubs of *Phyllophaga* beetles (May or June beetles) eat these eggs. Soon after, the worm embryo (the acanthor) hatches from the egg and uses its blade-like hooks to cut through the gut of the beetle larva. At this stage it is a parasite of the beetle larva, feeding and growing. The pig eats the infected beetle larvae to complete the cycle, becoming infective in 60–90 days.

**33 i.** False. Blood associated with hookworm infection is blackened because it is digested in the small intestine. Fresh blood would be seen in the faeces if infection had occurred in the large intestine.

**ii.** False. *Cheyletiella blakei* is the 'walking dandruff' mite of cats. This surface-dwelling mite prefers to reside on skin and in the hair coat. 'Walking dandruff' refers to debris from dermatitis that moves with the mites.

**iii.** False. This condition worsens with age.

**iv.** False. MLs act by binding to receptors on worm nerve cells, causing chloride channels to remain open so that there is a continuous flow of chloride ions through the nerve cell membrane. This flow of chloride ions prevents transmission of stimuli to the next nerve cell, causing the parasite to become paralyzed and die.

**v.** True. Because whipworms take 3 months to mature, this regimen will destroy the worms as they mature, prevent contamination of the environment and address reinfection.

**vi.** False. Lufenuron disrupts the synthesis and deposition of chitin by blocking the enzyme chitin synthetase, and chitin is necessary for the survival of eggs and larvae. Lufenuron has ovicidal and larvicidal activity, but no deleterious effects on adult fleas.

34 A 5-year-old female cat is presented with marked tremors, muscle fasciculations and hyperexcitability within 4 hours of spot application of a permethrin-based topical insecticide for fleas.
i. Are these clinical signs associated with exposure to the insecticide?
ii. Why are cats more prone to toxicity with permethrin products than other animal species?
iii. Name some other causes of seizures in cats.
iv. How would you manage this cat?
v. What advice would you give to the owner?

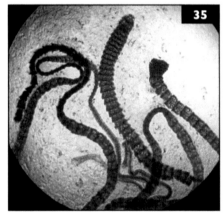

35 These organisms (35) were identified in the intestine of a juvenile gerbil during a post-mortem examination. The gerbil was one of a group displaying signs of diarrhoea, lethargy and ill thrift.
i. What is this organism?
ii. What is its significance?
iii. How would you treat the remaining gerbils?

**34 i.** Yes. Permethrin toxicity is a common cause of severe generalized tremors in cats. This can occur after some dog flea products are applied to cats.

**ii.** The specific reason for this increased sensitivity to permethrin is thought to be associated with a deficiency in glucuronidase, which is necessary for permethrin metabolism via glucuronidation. Additionally, the hydrolytic enzymes that degrade pyrethroid esters have a slow rate of hydrolysis in cats compared with other species, thus increasing their susceptibility.

**iii.** Hepatic encephalopathy, meningioma, lymphosarcoma (which may affect the CNS), feline infectious peritonitis (with meningitis or meningoencephalitis), intracranial intra-arachnoid cyst, hydrocephalus, insulin overdose, thiamine deficiency, *Toxoplasma gondii* intracranial cyst, *Cuterebra* larvae myiasis (causing feline ischaemic encephalopathy).

**iv.** Treatment is aimed at controlling seizures and tremors and administering supportive care. Diazepam can be used to control seizures or tremors. Gaseous anaesthesia may be necessary for refractory seizures. Once the cat has been stabilized it can be bathed in lukewarm water, with detergent to wash off residual insecticide. Intravenous fluids should be administered to maintain hydration.

**v.** Permethrin insecticides are very toxic to cats and are contraindicated in this species. Follow the manufacturer's instructions carefully and never give more than the dosage stated on the packet. Carefully monitor your cat after giving any flea/tick medication. Seek the advice of a veterinarian before using any flea or tick medication, especially over-the-counter products.

**35 i.** The dwarf tapeworm *Rodentolepis nana* (formerly *Hymenolepis nana*) or the rat tapeworm *Hymenolepis diminuta*. The two species can be morphologically differentiated, based on the size and shape of the eggs. Also, *R. nana* adults have an armed rostellum, whereas *H. diminuta* adults have no hooks on the scolex.

**ii.** These tapeworms are often asymptomatic; however, they may be associated with signs of debilitation, diarrhoea and dehydration, intestinal obstruction and death. Both are considered zoonotic.

**iii.** Praziquantel is considered effective.

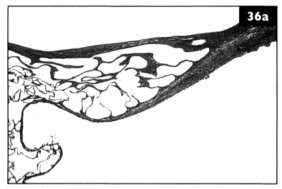

36 During the course of a routine post-mortem examination of a macaque monkey, small nodular lesions are detected in the lungs. Histological sections (36a) reveal morphological changes in the pulmonary parenchyma.

i. What are the features of these lesions?

ii. What is the cause of these lesions?

iii. Describe the life cycle of the associated organism.

iv. Is treatment advisable/feasible?

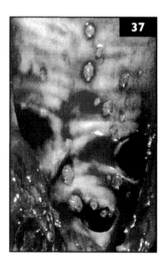

37 A 2-year-old male Border Collie presented with a dry cough, dyspnoea and stridor. An initial diagnosis of 'kennel cough' was made and the dog was treated with amoxicillin and prednisolone, which temporarily relieved the clinical signs, but signs recurred when medication was stopped. Further examination by direct endoscopy revealed multifocal raised submucosal masses in the caudal trachea and adjacent portions of mainstem bronchi (37). The masses contained slowly moving nematodes, some of which protruded and retracted from the nodules.

i. What is your diagnosis?

ii. Describe the life cycle of these nematodes.

iii. How should the dog be treated?

**36 i.** The lesions consist of bullae, or coalesced alveoli, many of which show a fibrous tissue reaction.

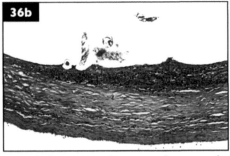

**ii.** Histological examination reveals portions of arthropod parasites (**36b**). These are typical of *Pneumonyssus* mites, which inhabit the respiratory system of certain taxa of primates.

**iii.** The life cycle takes place entirely in the lungs. It is believed that transmission is by direct contact because transmission to newborn monkeys can be prevented by isolating them from infected mothers. A nymphal stage has been reported in one species, *Pneumonyssus simicola*.

**iv.** Treatment is generally not recommended because dead mites can elicit a marked inflammatory/foreign body response, which may be deleterious to the monkey.

**37 i.** The presence of characteristic nodules at the tracheal bifurcation with intralesional nematodes strongly suggests *Filaroides (Oslerus) osleri*.

**ii.** *O. osleri* has a direct life cycle. Dogs are infected by ingestion of L1s through different routes: (1) puppies become infected with larvae from the saliva of their mother while she is licking or cleaning them; (2) dogs become infected by eating regurgitated food and ingesting larvae from infected faeces. Following infection, L1s penetrate the mucosa of the small intestine and migrate to the right side of the heart via lymphatics or the hepatic venous circulation and then to the lungs via pulmonary arteries. Maturation of larvae into adult worms triggers an inflammatory reaction inside the dog's respiratory tract, causing the formation of fibrotic tracheobronchial nodules. Adults reside in these nodules and the gravid females protrude their caudal end through the respiratory epithelium to lay embryonated eggs in the lumen. Many eggs hatch immediately, releasing L1s that are directly infectious. Eggs and larvae are coughed up and either expectorated in sputum or swallowed and voided in faeces.

**iii.** Fenbendazole (50 mg/kg for 10–26 days) controls the clinical signs and leads to resolution of tracheobronchial nodules. Oxfendazole (10 mg/kg/day for 28 days) gives the same efficacy. Regimens using ivermectin or doramectin (usually off-licence) provide a shorter treatment course. (**Note:** Ivermectin must be used with care in Collie-type dogs.)

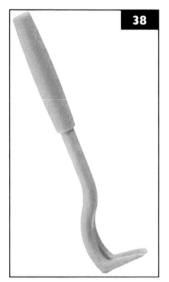

38 What is this instrument (38), and what is it used for?

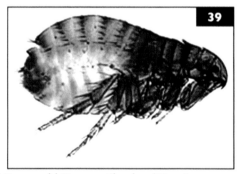

39 A very pruritic 10-year-old German Shepherd Dog is presented. On investigation you count 44 active fleas (39). The owner has not been using any flea prevention, but says she herself has developed some bites around her ankles.

i. If a client has a pre-existing household infestation of fleas, how long will it take to eradicate the infestation once correct treatment of the pet and household is initiated?

ii. What treatment/advice would you recommend?

iii. What is an insect growth regulator (IGR), and when would you use this?

38 A tick removal device. Ticks are irritating arthropods that prey on livestock and companion animals. They are excellent carriers and transmitters of many microbial diseases during the taking of a blood meal. The best method of controlling ticks and the diseases transmitted by them is through a combination of tick avoidance and using tick preventive medications. However, ticks can still be found attached to an animal's body. Therefore, finding and quickly removing them is important in reducing the risk of associated disease. Pets should be checked frequently for signs of ticks after coming back from a potential tick-infested area, even if already using tick prevention medications. Removing a tick is best done by using a commercially available tick removal device or a tweezers to pull it off. Grab the tick as close to the head as possible and with steady, gentle pressure, pull the tick out of the skin. Do not twist the tick – pull straight up and out. If the head of the tick remains in the skin, try to grab it and remove as much as possible. Wear gloves when removing a tick to minimize the chance of personal infection.

39 i. The pupal window period is usually 2–3 months. Because no insecticide kills the pupae, this is the time it takes to allow hatching of existing flea pupae in the environment, which will depend on temperature, relative humidity and availability of hosts. Pupae can lie dormant for up to 1 year if left undisturbed in colder climates.
ii. Minimum treatment involves: use of veterinary flea product on all pets in the household; spraying the entire house/car/caravan/shed with an IGR; increasing temperature and humidity within the home; washing bedding at 60°C; and vacuuming to stimulate pupal hatch. Explain to the client that she will continue to see fleas on her pets until all the pupae have hatched (for 2–3 months on average).
iii. IGRs act to inhibit development into the next immature life stage of an insect. For instance, they may impede rigidity of the flea egg tooth, preventing the larvae hatching from eggs (lufenuron), or may mimic juvenile growth hormone levels, which would normally drop to initiate the next life stage (s-methoprene). Spot-on formulations should be used in conjunction with an adulticide to prevent laying of viable eggs into the environment. Household spray formulations should be used during a household infestation to kill pre-existing eggs and larvae. An adulticide on the pet will prevent further infestation of the environment.

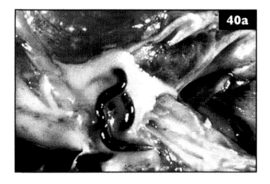

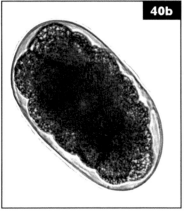

40 Individual pigs within groups of outdoor breeding pigs (2–3 years old) show poor body condition and some have noticeable blood in the urine. The pigs are raised in muddy, open-range conditions in an area with a semi-tropical climate and prolonged rainy seasons. At post-mortem examination of an older affected animal, multifocal fibrotic lesions are noted in the liver and dark thick nematodes are noted in the fat above the kidney (40a). Microscopical examination of urine sediment shows eggs (40b).
i. What is the name of these nematodes? Are they pathogenic?
ii. Discuss the nematode's life cycle. Why do these parasites occur only in warm damp climates?

41 List some of the problems associated with faecal egg counts.

**40 i.** *Stephanurus dentatus*, the pig kidney worm. Adult worms have a predilection for the walls of the ureter and capsules in the peri-renal fat. They are large-bodied worms (2–4 cm long) with a dark mottled appearance because the transparent cuticle shows the internal organs. Larvae cause severe damage, particularly in the liver, as they migrate throughout the body and they cause loss of appetite and body condition. Blood is often passed in the urine. There may be considerable muscle wastage.

**ii.** Adult females live in cysts in the kidney fat and ureters and pass eggs into the urine. Eggs develop into infective larvae in the environment in 2–7 days. The life cycle can be direct through the oral intake of infected larvae or by cutaneous penetration, or indirect through consumption of larvae-infected earthworms. After ingestion, larvae migrate from the intestine throughout the body (particularly the liver) over a period of 4–6 months before they finally arrive at the kidneys to mature. The cycle from egg to adult takes up to 1 year and females lay large numbers of eggs each day. Infection is more common in pigs raised outdoors in warm, temperate, subtropical and tropical regions because the pre-parasitic larvae are free living and may also utilize earthworms as transport hosts. Larvae die out quickly in cold, dry conditions.

**41** (1) The consistency of faecal material can influence egg counts; watery diarrhoea can cause a dilution effect, whereas very dry faeces or constipation can cause a relative concentration of parasite numbers.

(2) Eggs can be expelled from hosts at different rates throughout the day, therefore if following a group of animals over time, it is best to obtain each sample at a similar time of day.

(3) Eggs can be distributed unevenly throughout the sample and this is thought to be of particular issue in horse and cattle samples.

(4) Some parasites (e.g. *Fasciola hepatica*) have a natural intermittent shedding pattern of eggs, therefore the absence of eggs is not necessarily an indication of lack of parasites. Also, immature stages of parasites do not shed eggs, and in parasites where inhibition at an early stage of development is commonplace (e.g. with cyathostomins in horses or *Ostertagia ostertagi* in cattle), accurate determination of worm burdens can be very difficult at certain times of the year.

(5) A relaxation of immunity can occur around parturition in some hosts (particularly sheep) with an associated increase in parasite development or acquisition of new infections, with a resultant increase in egg counts.

(6) The McMaster technique commonly used has a detection limit of 50 epg, therefore improved sensitivity methods are needed to detect drug resistance in certain situations.

42 It is August in England and you are asked to evaluate a 7-year-old Thoroughbred-cross mare that was purchased 6 months ago. The horse has broken hairs, excessively flaky skin and thickening of the skin of the mane and tail (42a). The horse is constantly rubbing these regions and it also rolls excessively in the field and stable.

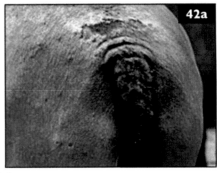

i. What is the differential diagnosis for these clinical signs?

ii. How would you confirm your diagnosis?

iii. How would you treat this case?

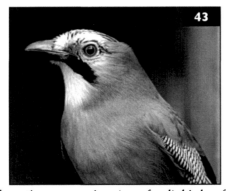

43 A collection of captive companion (non-food) birds of different species is affected by roundworms. One outdoor aviary hosts a colony of corvids used for ethological studies (43).

i. Would you treat all the different species of birds with the same anthelmintic drug?

ii. How do you choose the route of administration?

iii. How do you treat corvids without interfering with the behavioural experiments?

iv. How often would you monitor the endoparasite reinfection rate in outdoor aviaries hosting companion birds?

**42 i.** *Culicoides* hypersensitivity, the sucking louse *Haematopinus asini* and psoroptic mange cause pruritus affecting the mane. *H. asini, Oxyuris equi*, psoroptic mange and *Culicoides* hypersensitivity cause pruritus of the tail. *Culicoides* hypersensitivity (most likely in this case) is a common cause of pruritus in the horse. Always check for broken hairs and skin thickening

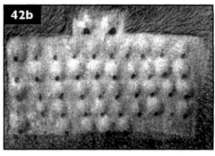

in the mane and tail at pre-purchase examinations. There may be a hereditary predisposition in some cases.

**ii.** History and clinical signs plus a skin scrape and biopsy of the affected area. Histopathological findings for *Culicoides* hypersensitivity include perivascular eosinophilic dermatitis with epidermal spongiosis, tissue necrosis and collagen degeneration. An intradermal skin reaction test (**42b**) is available.

**iii.** Reduce exposure to the *Culicoides* flies and manage the delayed hypersensitivity reaction to the saliva of the fly. Management of the overexuberant inflammatory response usually requires administration of oral steroids (problematic in animals that have other concurrent problems such as laminitis). Oral antihistamines can be used to manage mild to moderate pruritus.

**43 i.** Drugs commonly used in poultry might be toxic or associated with side-effects in some companion avian species. Before starting any treatment you should refer to an avian formulary for a review of the species-specific pharmacology and pharmacokinetics data, when available.

**ii.** The route is chosen according to several factors, such as the number of birds to be treated, the stress sensitivity of the avian host to handling procedures and the pharmacokinetics of the drug.

**iii.** Corvids are one of the most intelligent groups of birds. The parasitological treatment of birds used as a model for behavioural studies requires a different therapeutic approach because the choice of drug has to deal with the route of administration and the negative emotional effects of bird handling. Handling and stressful clinical procedures should be avoided if possible.

**iv.** Direct contact with wild birds, availability of invertebrates as paratenic or IHs and the natural ground increase the frequency of reinfection. Seasonality should also be taken into account; parasite burdens grow quicker during the hot season and birds living in outdoor aviaries can be reinfected in a relatively short period (1–2 months), therefore the frequency of parasitological screening should be higher during summer and autumn.

**44** What advice would you give to the owner of the horse described in case **42** in terms of long-term management?

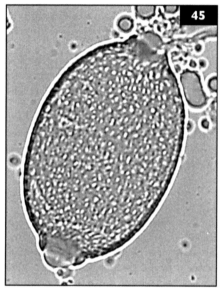

**45** You perform a routine faecal examination on a captive-bred kestrel and find eggs such as the one shown (**45**).
**i.** Identify the egg.
**ii.** How would you treat this parasitic infection?
**iii.** What control measures would you implement to prevent this infection?

44 Several factors can be used to manage horses with *Culicoides* hypersensitivity, mainly involving reducing exposure to the flies:

- *Culicoides* species prefer stagnant water, damp soil and warm, decaying vegetation for completion of their life cycle. Therefore, wet fields should be avoided and breezier areas sought as they will be less popular for the flies. Avoid areas with still water and make sure that areas of rotting vegetation are removed. These include muck heaps, poached land and areas of old forage.
- *Culicoides* flies prefer to feed at dusk and dawn, therefore it is worth stabling horses at these times to limit exposure to the flies. If possible, close stable doors and windows.
- Fans within the stable create a less favourable environment for the fly. Insect repellents or insecticides are sometimes useful. Insecticides include daily application of benzyl benzoate to susceptible areas, or permethrin and related compounds, which tend to have longer-lasting effects.
- Boett blankets and hoods are very effective in preventing fly bites and can be used long term. The blankets must be well-fitting and not have any holes in them. Ideally, horses should be wearing the rugs as a preventive measure prior to developing clinical signs.

45 i. *Capillaria* species.

ii. *Capillaria* parasites often demonstrate multiple drug tolerance to levamisole, avermectins and standard doses of fenbendazole. Fenbendazole (20–25 mg/kg PO q24h for 5 days) appears to be most efficacious. Ivermectin (0.5–1 mg/kg PO once) may also be effective. Repeat faecal testing is recommended 3–4 weeks after treatment to confirm successful treatment.

iii. *Capillaria* species usually have a direct life cycle, but may use earthworms as IHs. For successful parasite control, environmental decontamination and preventing access to IHs is essential. This may be achieved by using concrete floors or impermeable membranes covered with non-contaminated substrate. Faecal screening should be performed twice yearly.

46 A 2-year-old Standardbred stallion is presented for stumbling and falling twice in the past week. In addition, the horse's appetite has decreased over the past 5 days and he seems 'unsteady' on his hindlimbs. Physical examination reveals slight wear on the dorsum of the toe of each hind hoof. There is moderate gluteal muscle atrophy on the right side, while the left gluteal muscle mass is normal (46). The gait is evaluated at a walk and at a trot, and the horse's movements are evaluated

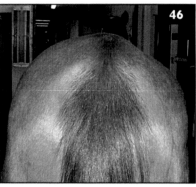

when he is circled in wide and tight circles to the left and to the right. Weakness, ataxia, dysmetria and spasticity are graded on a scale of 0 (normal) to 4+ (severely abnormal), and results are as follows:

| Weakness | Forelimbs, 2+ | Right hindlimb, 3+; Left hindlimb, 2+ |
| --- | --- | --- |
| Ataxia | Forelimbs, 1+ | Hindlimbs, 2+ |
| Spasticity | Forelimbs, 1+ | Right hindlimb, 2+; Left hindlimb, 1+ |
| Dysmetria | Forelimbs, 1+ | Right hindlimb, 2+; Left hindlimb, 1+ |

1+ = manipulative tests are necessary in order to detect a deficit; 2+ = deficit detectable at a walk or trot, but subtle; 3+ = deficit detectable at a walk or trot, but obvious; 4+ = the horse is in danger of falling because of a severe deficit.

The 'sway response' to pushing laterally, to the right and to the left, against the shoulders is normal. The sway response to pulling laterally on the tail reveals less resistance when pulled to the right than when pulled to the left.
i. Based on the physical and neurological examination findings, where anatomically is this horse's problem?
ii. What is the 'sway response', and what does it evaluate?
iii. What diseases should be considered in your differential diagnosis?

47 What is 'hypobiosis'? Which parasite species of ruminants use this phenomenon? Can this condition be managed with anthelmintics?

**46 i.** Neurological deficits in all four limbs and no cranial nerve abnormalities implies a lesion in the C1/C5 portion of the spinal cord. Also, gluteal muscle atrophy suggests a lower motor neuron (ventral horn grey matter) lesion in the lumbosacral spinal cord (L6/S2) or the motor nerves supplying the gluteal muscles (cranial and caudal gluteal nerves).
**ii.** It checks for weakness and ataxia and helps to assess the symmetry of neurological signs; normally, one can pull a horse 30% off midline with the tail pull.
**iii.** Equine protozoal myeloencephalitis (EPM) caused by the protozoan parasite *Sarcocystis neurona*, cervical vertebral stenotic myelopathy (CVSM, wobbler syndrome), traumatic injury (e.g. vertebral fracture, subluxation), equine herpesvirus type 1 myelopathy, West Nile virus infection and equine degenerative myelopathy (EDM). Clinical signs for CVSM and EDM are usually symmetric. Eastern equine encephalitis (EEE) virus infection would be unlikely based on the relatively long duration of clinical signs. The presence of gluteal muscle atrophy implies 'lower motor neuron' spinal cord involvement, which is common in EPM, but less likely in all other differentials.

**47** 'Hypobiosis' is the term used to describe the arrested development of nematode parasites inside host animals. This phenomenon enables parasites to survive in their host in a dormant state during adverse conditions that may otherwise kill the parasite or prevent its progeny from surviving in the external environment. Therefore, larvae tend to become dormant as a response to host immunity (which is parasite-specific) or to seasonal conditions (e.g. 'summer' inhibition in response to dry summer conditions or 'winter' inhibition in more temperate climates). Many important nematode species (e.g. *Haemonchus contortus*, *Teladorsagia* and *Dictyocaulus*) undergo hypobiosis. Other nematodes (e.g. *Trichostrongylus* species, *Chabertia ovina* and *Oesophagostomum venulosum*) are also likely to enter an arrested state. Levamisole, benzimidazoles and MLs have killing activity against the inhibited stages of *H. contortus* and *Teladorsagia* spp., although this is variable for levamisole. The new anthelmintic monepantel recorded high efficacy against the inhibited fourth-stage larvae of *H. contortus* and *Teladorsagia* species at all locations within the abomasum when administered orally to sheep at 2.5 mg/kg.

48 An adult fish is presented with rapid gilling behaviour and gasping. Wet mount preparations made of scrapings of the body and gill surfaces reveal active parasites that move in a jerky manner. The parasites are fixed and stained (48).
i. What are these parasites, and where do they live?
ii. What are the major types of these parasites?
iii. Can infection with these parasites be fatal to the fish?
iv. How should this fish be treated?

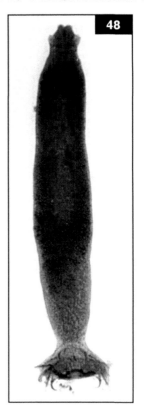

49 During examination of an injured wild tawny owl, several flies (49) are found crawling among the plumage.
i. What are these flies?
ii. What is its significance?
iii. What treatment would you advise?

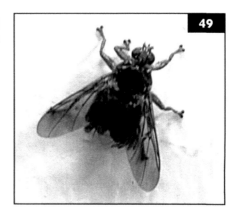

**48 i.** Monogeneans, single-host flatworms (flukes) that are very common in marine water and freshwater fish. They live mainly on the skin and gills of affected fish, but a few species can be found on the eye, in the body cavity and in ureters. In freshwater fish, the primary species seen are *Dactylogyrus* (gill fluke) and *Gyrodactylus* (skin fluke); however, either can be located on the skin and gills.

**ii.** *Dactylogyrus* flukes are egg layers (oviparous); *Gyrodactylus* flukes are embryo bearing (viviparous). Oviparous monogeneans release eggs into the water, which hatch into a free-swimming stage (oncomiracidium) that seeks out a fish host. Viviparous monogeneans release live larvae that are immediately parasitic. *Dactylogyrus* can be recognized by the prominent 2–4 anterior eyespots and a four-pointed anterior end (**48**). Gyrodactylids have no eyespots and often have an embryo visible inside the fluke (see **11**).

**iii.** Yes. Monogenean-infected fish will exhibit flashing, rubbing, gasping, lethargy, clamped fins, excess mucus production, secondary cutaneous ulcerations, scale loss and death in severe infections.

**iv.** Affected fish should be quarantined and treated with 2 ppm praziquantel for 3 days. Other treatments include organophosphates, formalin, potassium permanganate and mebendazole.

**49 i.** Hippoboscid flies, otherwise known as louse or flat flies.

**ii.** Hippoboscid flies are common on many owls, but are generally considered to be non-pathogenic. However, they can cause blood loss and anaemia and are potential vectors for a variety of pathogens including *Leucocytozoon* species, *Haemoproteus* species and poxvirus.

**iii.** Fipronil spray (3 ml/kg) applied under each wing is effective.

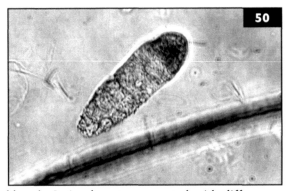

50 A 3-year-old male Syrian hamster presented with diffuse generalized scaling and alopecia, as well as a poor appetite and lethargy. A distended abdomen was palpated and on ballottement there was a fluid thrill. Microscopical examination of a scrape from the skin lesion revealed this organism (50).
i. What is your diagnosis?
ii. How do you confirm the diagnosis?
iii. What is your differential diagnosis?
iv. How can this problem be managed?

51 Equine protozoal myeloencephalitis is diagnosed in the horse in case **46**.
i. What parasite causes this disease, and how is the infection acquired by horses?
ii. What tests are available for the diagnosis of this infection? What is the basis of each type of test?

**50 i.** Demodicosis. This animal also had epitheliotropic lymphoma of the skin and lymphoma in the abdomen.
**ii.** Examination of plucked hair or a skin biopsy.
**iii.** *Demodex aurati* and *D. criceti* infestation. There is often an underlying condition such as malnutrition, neoplasia or intercurrent infection. *D. aurati* is found in hair follicles with minimal inflammation, whereas *D. criceti* is usually present in epidermal pits. There is no evidence of spread between hamsters. *Notoedres notoedres* and *N. cati* have occasionally been reported on the ears, nose, feet and perineal areas. Dermatophytosis and hyperadrenocorticism are rarely reported in hamsters. Allergic dermatitis is recognized by some authors. Hamster polyoma virus infection is a consideration, as some hamster colonies are affected by this cutaneous neoplastic disease associated with viral infection.
**iv.** Establish the underlying cause of the demodicosis and remove if possible. There are no effective treatments for hyperadrenocorticism or lymphoma. Old hamsters with extensive demodicosis, which is a marker for underlying disease, are frequently euthanized. However, some normal hamsters may be seen with many *Demodex* mites, therefore check the diet and husbandry. There are various protocols for the use of amitraz (e.g. 0.025% dips every week for several weeks), but this treatment can be fatal.

**51 i.** *Sarcocystis neurona*, a protozoan parasite. The opossum is the definitive natural host for this organism. Horses are accidental hosts, becoming infected following ingestion of feed or water contaminated with *S. neurona* sporocysts in opossum faeces.
**ii.** The most commonly used test is Western blot analysis for antibodies to certain antigens on the protozoan (16-kDa and 30-kDa proteins). The test can be run on serum or CSF. However, a high percentage of horses are seropositive, which indicates only exposure to the agent and not necessarily CNS infection, so a positive result on CSF is more meaningful. A PCR-based test was developed several years ago to detect *S. neurona* DNA in CSF. However, this test is rarely used because of the high number of false-negative results. Both tests therefore have limitations and results should be interpreted in combination with neurological examination findings, clinical history and other diagnostic findings. Currently, definitive diagnosis of EPM is by identifying the protozoan in nervous tissue (histopathology or culture from fresh tissue) at necropsy.

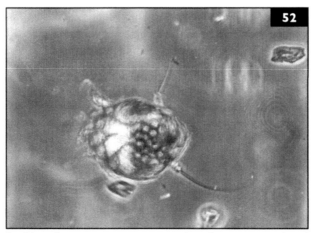

52 A 3-month-old male guinea pig is presented with pruritus and multifocal small areas of alopecia over the trunk. This organism (52) is found in a skin scrape.
i. What is your diagnosis?
ii. How would you confirm the diagnosis?
iii. What is the differential diagnosis?
iv. How would you treat this guinea pig?
v. Is there any zoonotic potential?

# 52: Answer

52 i. *Trixacarus caviae*. Dermatophytosis was also detected.

ii. A hair pluck may identify this mange mite.

iii. *T. caviae* infestation; dermatophytosis (*Trichophyton mentagrophytes*) (normal in up to 13.3% of guinea pigs) starting at the head and spreading to the dorsal lumbar area; inflammation associated with an allergic response to fungal elements; *Malassezia ovale* has been reported to cause skin lesions; lice infestation (*Gliricola porcelli, Gyropus ovalis*) usually does not cause major problems – they are obligate parasites but may survive in the bedding; vitamin C deficiency – inappropriate diet or secondary to other debilitating conditions; *Chirodiscoides caviae* (fur mite), *Sarcoptes scabiei, Notoedres muris, Myocoptes* and *Demodex caviae* are uncommon to rare; alopecia associated with aggression, intense breeding, weaning, (self-) barbering or ovarian imbalance – may be associated with diffuse alopecia; fleas, especially if a multipet household and guinea pig allowed into communal areas.

iv. Ivermectin (0.4 mg/kg SC or PO every 10 days for 3 treatments). Establish appropriate diet formulation: ensure fresh good quality guinea pig pellet food and hay, fresh cabbage, parsley, spinach, red and green peppers, broccoli, tomatoes, kiwi fruit, kale and oranges. Daily supplementation of drinking water with vitamin C (200 mg to 1 g/l). Plenty of fresh water. Fungal infections: consider bathing with chlorhexidine and miconazole shampoos. Oral itraconazole has been recommended (5 mg/kg q24h for 14 days).

v. *T. caviae* can cause a transient skin problem for humans in contact with an affected guinea pig. Dermatophytosis may also be a potential zoonosis.

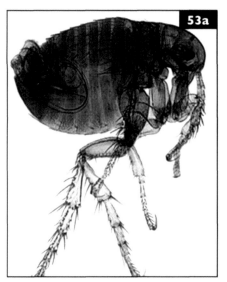

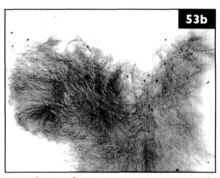

53 Flea infestation is a commonly encountered problem in companion animals (53a).

i. If you want to control a flea problem, what parts of the flea life cycle should you target, and with what types of drugs or chemicals?

ii. What is the connection between a flea infestation and a tapeworm infection?

iii. Apart from finding adult fleas on a cat or dog, the presence of 'flea dirt' is also considered a definitive diagnosis of an infestation. What is flea dirt (53b)?

iv. Are companion animal fleas hazardous to humans?

v. Why is it important to treat both the surrounding environment and the pet during a flea infestation?

54 A flock of finches has a history of diarrhoea, weight loss and sensory depression. Young birds seem to be more affected than older birds, and the mortality rate is higher in young birds. Gross necropsy reveals hyperaemia and thickening of the intestinal wall. Fresh smears of the intestinal content show the presence of these tiny round organisms (54).

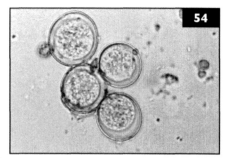

i. Identify these parasites.

ii. Are they important in avian medicine?

iii. Which bird families are most affected by these parasites?

iv. How do birds become infected?

**53 i.** Adult fleas with an adulticide and/ or environmental stages with either sprays with insecticidal or IGR activity or by relying on newly emerged fleas being killed once they have located a suitable treated host.

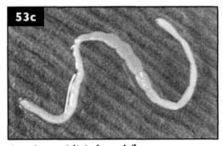

**ii.** The tapeworm *Dipylidium caninum* (53c) uses fleas and chewing lice as an IH. Cats or dogs are infected with tapeworms when they ingest tapeworm larvae (cysticercoid)-infected fleas.

**iii.** Flea faeces.

**iv.** Yes, fleas can bite humans and some individuals become hypersensitive.

**v.** By the time the owner notices a flea infestation there can be a large number of immature fleas in the environment. Stages in the environment may be controlled by insecticidal treatment of the host (e.g. treated dander falling into the environment) or by direct treatment of the environment.

**54 i.** Unsporulated oocysts of *Isospora* species, a single-cell coccidian protozoan parasite.

**ii.** Coccidiosis is one of the most serious diseases of poultry and companion birds. Most of the coccidian families are intracellular parasites of the epithelial cells of the vertebrate intestine.

**iii.** All bird species can be infected by coccidia, although some avian families (e.g. finches, canaries, galliformes, falconiformes, columbiformes and some psittaciformes) seem to be particularly sensitive to coccidian infection.

**iv.** By direct transmission. Birds ingest food or water contaminated by faecal material containing the infective sporulated oocysts. Under natural conditions birds are repeatedly exposed to small numbers of oocysts and so develop some protective immunity. However, intensive farming conditions and stressful events such as transportation and high bird density, along with conditions that permit the build-up of infective oocysts in the environment, can lead to the development of overt disease.

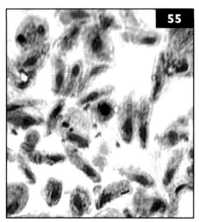

55 A 7-month-old male kitten is presented with chronic diarrhoea and poor body condition. The perineum and hindlimbs are stained with a yellow faecal material. Motile, flagellated trophozoites (55) of trichomonads, featuring a pear-shaped body with an undulating membrane and three free anterior flagella, are visible on direct microscopical examination of a rectal faecal swab.

i. What is your diagnosis?

ii. How do cats become infected with this parasite, and what are the risk factors for infection?

iii. What other laboratory tests are required to confirm this infection?

iv. How can this infection be treated?

v. Can this parasite infect people?

**55 i.** Feline intestinal tritrichomonosis, caused by the protozoan *Tritrichomonas foetus*, which has recently attracted attention as a cause of chronic large-bowel diarrhoea.

**ii.** Transmission from cat to cat is by the faecal–oral route. The disease is mainly seen in densely housed young cats (i.e. where faecal–oral transmission may readily occur). Cats living in multicat households (catteries or shelters) are at high risk of infection. Young, pedigree cats in high-density housing appear to be most susceptible to infection.

**iii.** Microscopical examination of wet mounts of freshly voided faeces, faecal culture in selective media (e.g. InPouch™, TF-Feline medium), colonic/ileal biopsy and immunohistochemistry or PCR-based assays using species-specific primers. This should form part of the routine work-up of chronic diarrhoea in cats, particularly in young purebred cats and cats with large-bowel diarrhoea.

**iv.** Fenbendazole (50 mg/kg q24h for 5 days) with metronidazole (10 mg/kg q12h) may be effective. Tritrichomonosis can be successfully treated with ronidazole (30–50 mg/kg q12–24h for 14 days); the use of this drug is off-label and close monitoring is mandatory because cats treated with high doses may exhibit neurological signs. Also, reduce environmental stress, optimize litter tray hygiene and treat or isolate in-contact cats, which may be a source of reinfection.

**v.** Yes. People in contact with infected cats are advised to take basic hygiene precautions to avoid ingesting the parasite. Cat scratches or bites should always be washed immediately with soap and water. Anyone with a weakened immune system should not handle cat faeces or litter boxes.

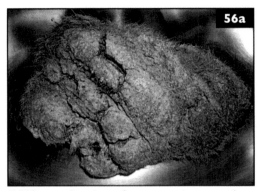

56 You are the wildlife veterinarian of a mountain natural reserve that hosts a large population of ungulates, including ibex, chamois and deer. An adult chamois is found dead inside the reserve near the end of winter. The animal shows severe chronic lesions on the face, ears, trunk, abdomen and limbs. The skin is very thickened and heavily encrusted, with fissuring (56a).
i. Given the pathological findings, what is the most likely aetiology of this condition?
ii. What laboratory tests can be used to confirm the diagnosis?
iii. If you want to carry out a serological survey to determine the prevalence of infection, what factors should be considered in sampling the chamois herd?
iv. How should this condition be managed in a wild naïve ungulate population?

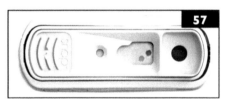

57 This is a patient-side SNAP *Giardia* Test kit designed for use with dog and cat faeces (57).
i. What is the kit specifically detecting in an animal's faeces?
ii. What other tests are available for diagnosis of giardiosis?
iii. How reliable is a positive SNAP *Giardia* test result?
iv. Is giardiosis in dogs and cats considered zoonotic?

**56 i.** Sarcoptic mange, one of the most severe parasitic diseases in chamois, with high mortality rates in naïve populations.

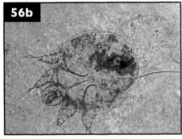

**ii.** Microscopical identification of the mites (56b) in deep skin scrapings. A diagnostic ELISA has been developed.

**iii.** To be epidemiologically significant, the sample size should be calculated based on the estimated/known prevalence of infection and the population size. For example, if a reserve hosts a population of 2,000 chamois and the estimated prevalence, based on available data from the closest infected area, is 5%, the lowest sample size needed to exclude the presence of the disease within the natural reserve is 58. Several free online software programs are available to calculate the size of the sample and other useful epidemiological parameters.

**iv.** In stable, wild ungulate populations, sarcoptic mange epizootics usually run their course. Although naïve populations suffer a high mortality rate the first time they are exposed to the mite, they usually recover fast. Later epizootics occurring after intervals of 10–15 years show a lower mortality rate, which is frequently confused with normal winter mortality. In some cases (e.g. captive ungulate collections or endangered populations) treatment with avermectin may be suggested.

**57 i.** The test is a rapid enzyme immunoassay for detecting *Giardia* antigen in canine and feline faeces. Positive results indicate the presence of antigen of *Giardia* trophozoites or cysts in the intestine.

**ii.** Detection of *Giardia* cysts and occasionally trophozoites in the faeces of affected animals. However, giardiosis is often difficult to diagnose because many of the signs are non-specific and because of the low sensitivity of microscopical methods (e.g. examination of faecal smears or flotation materials). This is due to the small size and low numbers of cysts present in the faeces and the intermittent shedding of these cysts.

**iii.** The sensitivity of the test is 95% and the specificity 99% compared with immunofluorescence microscopy, and 85% and 100%, respectively, compared with faecal floatation. The advantage of this test kit is that it permits the diagnosis of giardiosis in dogs and cats without special equipment and avoids the difficulties associated with flotation and microscopy.

**iv.** Up to 50% of infected dogs and cats are believed to shed zoonotic genotypes. Therefore, diagnosis and treatment of giardiosis in animals is important not only to eliminate clinical signs, but also to prevent transmission to other animals and humans.

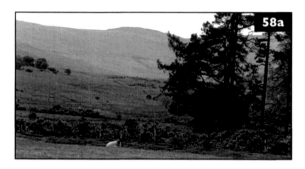

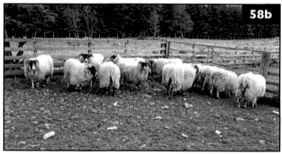

58 About 500 Scottish Blackface ewes are kept on an upland and hill farm in the southeast of Scotland. The ewes are routinely scanned for pregnancy via ultrasonography in early March. Those with twin lambs are kept in upland fields and those with single lambs are returned to the hill (58a). The flock is routinely vaccinated against chlamydial abortion and toxoplasmosis. During May, 49 of 300 ewes that had been scanned as pregnant with single lambs are identified as being barren (58b). Several abortions have been noted, especially in younger ewes, and there is evidence of scours in several ewes. A similar problem has occurred occasionally in recent years. Laboratory examination of aborted fetuses and placentae has indicated diagnoses of toxoplasmosis, chlamydial abortion, salmonellosis and campylobacteriosis in individual submissions, but has not identified a consistent cause of the flock's problem. No abortion or barren ewe problem has occurred in the animals scanned as pregnant with twin lambs.

i. How should this problem be further investigated?

ii. What is 'tick-borne fever'?

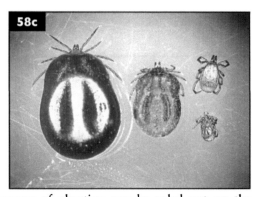

58 i. Common causes of abortion can be ruled out on the basis of clinical presentation, vaccination history and laboratory investigation results. The fact that the problem only occurred in ewes that were returned to the hill after scanning is significant, introducing the unlikely possibility of deficiency or toxicity diseases and the more likely involvement of tick-borne fever. The manner in which the hill had been grazed could have created an ideal *Ixodes ricinus* habitat and the opportunity for early spring infestation of ewes. The farmer had seen ticks (58c) on the faces of sheep grazing on the hill in the past, and the weather during March and April had been mild enough for questing to have occurred during those years when the problem had occurred, but had been too cold during problem-free years.
ii. An infection of sheep WBCs caused by the rickettsial agent *Anaplasma phagocytophilium*, which is transmitted by regurgitation of tick gut contents during blood feeding. The entire nymph and adult *I. ricinus* population on the farm may be affected, having acquired infection while feeding as larvae or nymphs on infected hosts. Infection of WBCs causes neutropenia, lymphopenia and thrombocytopenia, usually accompanied by a high fever lasting for up to 3 weeks, and is an important cause of abortion in naïve ewes.

**59 i.** How can a diagnosis of tick-borne fever be confirmed in the ewes described in case 58?
**ii.** How can abortions due to tick-borne fever be avoided in future years?

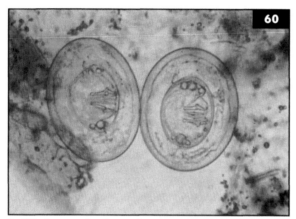

**60** These two *Raillietina* species (cestode or tapeworm) eggs (**60**) are found during a routine parasitological survey of a zoological collection of birds. Indoor and outdoor aviaries host different species of birds, according to their temperature needs.
**i.** What are the pathognomonic signs in birds affected by this parasite?
**ii.** What is the clinical significance of tapeworms in birds?
**iii.** Is one more likely to find avian tapeworm infection in indoor or in outdoor aviaries?

**59 i.** On knowledge of tick activity, confirmed by haematological findings of leucopenia and thrombocytopenia and demonstration of *A. phagocytophilium* inclusion bodies in cytoplasmic vacuoles of monocytes and neutrophils in Giemsa-stained blood smears. However, these are only seen during or shortly after the initial infection and are seldom useful for retrospective diagnosis of the cause of high barren or abortion rates. In this case diagnosis was suspected on the basis of neutropenia in 5/7 barren ewes, supported by serological identification of high *A. phagocytophilium* antibody titres in 6/6 barren ewes that were sampled.
**ii.** By controlling *I. ricinus* populations. Control by management of the environment is generally impractical, uneconomic or environmentally insensitive. Avoidance strategies can reduce the risk of vector-borne diseases, but need to be permanent because they only lead to a reduction in tick numbers when few alternative tick hosts are present. Most farmers rely on the use of acaricides to prevent infestation of their sheep. Plunge dipping of late-pregnant ewes is generally considered to be impractical. Deltamethrin and high cis cypermethrin pour-ons do not afford significant levels of persistent activity against *I. ricinus*, while alphacypermethrin affords 8–12 weeks' protection against reinfection. Options currently available for prevention of abortions caused by tick-borne fever are to avoid grazing the hill with pregnant ewes or to apply an alphacypermethrin pour-on drug to the single-bearing ewes at scanning time. The latter strategy may not prove to be wholly effective, because the highest concentrations of the pyrethroid drug are in the fleeced areas of the skin, rather than on hair-covered parts favoured by *I. ricinus* ticks.

**60 i.** Very frequently, avian tapeworm infections are asymptomatic, although some birds show diarrhoea, weight loss, eosinophilia and, rarely, fatal intestinal impaction due to a large number of adult parasites.
**ii.** This aspect is quite controversial because the pathogenicity of tapeworms differs according to the different avian goups/families and age classes. Young birds are more sensitive than adults to tapeworm infection and some families seem to show a higher prevalence of infection. The negative impact of tapeworms on avian health is probably underestimated because of the lack of specific signs and the low or inconsistent number of eggs/proglottids excreted in the faecal drops (intermittent shedding).
**iii.** Cestodes have an indirect life cycle and they need an invertebrate IH for completion of their life cycle. For example, *Raillietina* species use ants as an IH. Therefore, aviary birds housed on natural ground outdoors have easier access to IHs and a higher risk of tapeworm infection.

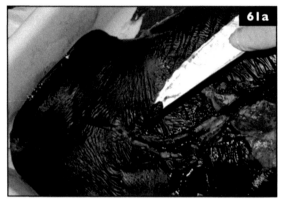

61 A 4-year-old Greyface ewe is submitted for post-mortem examination following sudden death. The carcass is in a poor condition and shows pale discolouration of the mucosa, a distended abdominal cavity and areas of wool loss. Examination of the liver reveals the presence of these abnormal structures (**61a**).
i. What is your diagnosis?
ii. How do sheep become infected with this parasite?
iii. How do you confirm the diagnosis?
iv. What advice would you offer to prevent this infection?

62 In late summer, one of six 8-month-old foals has nasal discharge. The anamnesis indicates that all six foals have access to the same paddock and they were dewormed once at 2 months old, but the owner cannot recall what product was used. A routine faecal examination is performed, and three of the six foals are found to be positive for *Parascaris* (epg 50, 150 and >1,000). All the foals are treated with generic ivermectin and re-examined 4 weeks later; the faeces of one foal still contains *Parascaris* eggs.
i. What is the explanation for the continued parasite problem despite treatment?
ii. How would you manage this problem?

**61 i.** Fasciolosis, caused by liver flukes of the genus *Fasciola*.

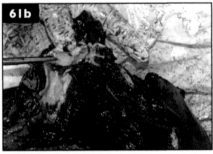

**ii.** By ingestion of infective larvae (encysted metacercariae). Juvenile forms excyst in the intestine, burrow through the gut wall, migrate across the peritoneal cavity and penetrate the liver parenchyma until they enter the bile ducts.

**iii.** Post-mortem examination reveals liver damage and flukes in the bile ducts (**61b**).

Faecal examination reveals fluke eggs. In live animals, glutamate dehydrogenase values are typically 10–20 times normal and remain elevated for several weeks even after treatment. Albumin concentrations are low (20 g/l [28–35 g/l]); globulin concentrations are elevated (>60 g/l [35–45 g/l]). Immunological tests have been developed to detect specific antibodies in the serum, and some can be used in milk samples.

**iv.** Administer anthelmintics to suppress fluke egg output and pasture metacercarial challenge. Improve drainage to reduce the rate of egg hatching and survival of free-living stages of flukes and prevent the establishment of snail populations. Grazing management to avoid contact between metacercariae and susceptible final hosts. Risk of resistance may be reduced by ensuring the correct drug dose is administered, using different drugs at strategic times and avoiding unnecessary treatment. Quarantine treatment of introduced animals using a sequentially administered combination of a benzimidazole and a salicylanilide derivative (or clorsulon in cattle) will reduce the spread of resistant flukes into new areas.

**62 i.** There is treatment failure, probably due to one or more of the following reasons: (1) incorrect administration; (2) expired anthelmintic drug; (3) slow mode of action of ivermectin against *P. equorum*, which is known as the dose-limiting species of equine nematodes for most broad-spectrum equine anthelmintics; it can take several days after treatment before the worms are killed; (4) lower quality of 'generic' ivermectins versus 'quality-brand' ivermectins; (5) presence of ivermectin-resistant *P. equorum* on the farm, as there are increasing reports in several countries of failure of ivermectin treatment against *P. equorum*; (6) there is no reduced treatment efficacy, and the eggs observed in the faeces are due to coprophagy, slow washout of eggs after treatment or single surviving worms because of resistance or the dose-limiting nature of the drug.

**ii.** Use a brand-name ivermectin or another ML, or use a benzimidazole, as they are known to have a high efficacy against ascarids. Follow-up on the efficacy, preferably 2 weeks after treatment.

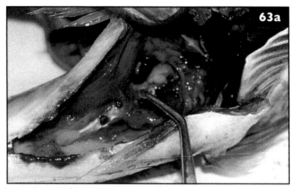

**63** This parasite (**63a**, in forceps) is seen during routine inspection of a fish used for feeding dolphins at a zoological garden.
i. What is this parasite?
ii. How do fish acquire them?
iii. What is their clinical significance?
iv. Can humans become infected?

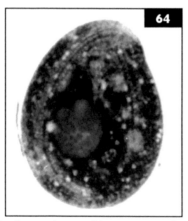

**64** This organism (**64**) is observed on a skin scraping taken from a goldfish.
i. What is it, and what is its significance?
ii. What treatment might be given?

63 i. L3 of the nematode parasite *Anisakis simplex*. They have a coiled filiform appearance (63b) and are normally observed in the body cavity, on the liver or stomach and, less frequently, in muscle.

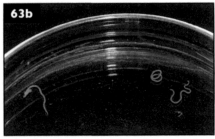

ii. *Anisakis* cycle in three hosts. Worms develop into adults in the gastric mucosa of the definitive host (dolphins, other marine mammals). Eggs are then released and passed in the faeces. In seawater, the eggs mature into L1s and then to free-living L2s. These are ingested by small crustaceans (first IH) in which the parasite matures into L3s, which are subsequently consumed by marine fish or squid (second IH). L3s migrate into the viscera and peritoneal cavity of the second IH. Ultimately, ingestion of infected fish by a marine mammal leads to development of L4s and then adults.

iii. Infected fish exhibit no external abnormalities. However, larvae of these nematodes are a major problem for commercial fishing industries. Infected marine animals exhibit ulcers, pain and bleeding. Fish used in feeding marine mammals must not be fed raw. Heating or freezing to –20°C (–4°F) for 24 hours is effective in killing the parasite.

iv. Yes, by consumption of raw or inadequately cooked infected marine fish or squid. This disease occurs where such dietary customs are practised (e.g. Japan, coastal regions of Europe, the USA). Live parasites penetrate the gut wall and cause acute gastroenteritis, abdominal pain, nausea and vomiting.

64 i. *Chilodenella* species, a mobile ciliate protozoan that infects the skin and gills of fish. Most *Chilodenella* species are free living, but a few species are pathogenic to fish. Some free-living species can cause damage in weakened fish in polluted waters, especially if the fish are stressed. Chilodenellosis is insidious and severe damage can occur before gross pathology is evident. Damage is mainly caused by the feeding activities of the parasites. They penetrate the host cell epidermis with their cytostome and suck out the contents of the epithelium. This feeding elicits strong cellular responses. In advanced stages there will be skin ulcers and secondary bacterial infections and mortalities.

ii. Formalin bath; formalin prolonged immersion; potassium permanganate prolonged immersion; copper prolonged immersion. Drugs should be used as part of an integrated health management strategy to mitigate the losses.

65 A 15-month-old male neutered DSH cat dies under anaesthesia during an elective surgical procedure. The cause of death is respiratory insufficiency due to severe pneumonia. Multiple types of parasitic larvae and eggs (65) are identified on histopathological examination of lung tissue.

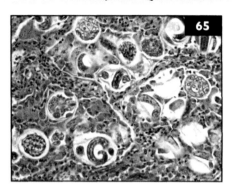

i. What is your diagnosis and differential diagnosis?
ii. How do cats become infected with this parasite?
iii. Why are some cats more prone to this disease than others?

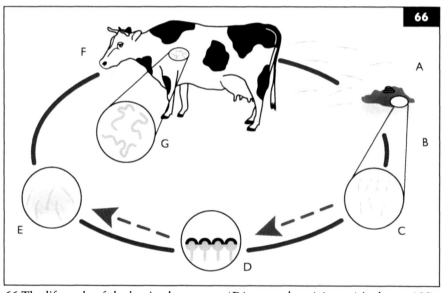

66 The life cycle of the bovine lungworm (*Dictyocaulus viviparus*) is shown (66).
i. Name and describe each of the lettered stages in the life cycle.
ii. What is the role of *Pilobolus* fungi in the life cycle?
iii. Why has the infection rate with this parasite in yearling and adult cattle been rising in some countries?
iv. Why is it necessary periodically to repeat faecal testing or perform serological testing to diagnose lungworm infection?

**65 i.** Aelurostrongylosis, casued by the lungworm *Aelurostrongylus abstrusus*. Differentials are other cardiorespiratory diseases of cats including parasitosis (e.g. *Dirofilaria immitis* or *Eucoleus aerophilus*), metastatic neoplasia, mycotic disease, chronic bacterial bronchitis, feline allergic bronchitis and tuberculosis. Baermann technique can be used to detect the larvae in faecal samples. CT scanning may be useful to differentiate aelurostrongylosis from other diseases with similar clinical signs.

**ii.** Adult worms live in the terminal bronchioles and alveolar ducts of the definitive host (cats) and, after mating, the gravid females deposit eggs that hatch into L1s. These pass up the bronchial escalator, are swallowed and released via faeces into the environment to continue their life cycle in a variety of slug and snail species. Cats become infected by ingesting the intermediate or paratenic (e.g. rodents, frogs, lizards, snakes, birds) hosts. After ingestion, the larvae migrate to the lungs via the blood and lymphatic vessels and evolve into adult stages, which reach sexual maturity after approximately 6 weeks post infection.

**iii.** Outdoor lifestyle: cats living outdoors (strays or owned but free ranging) become infected by preying on intermediate and/or paratenic hosts harbouring infective stages. Young age: kittens <1 year are 70% more likely to become infected due to the higher preying instinct of young animals.

**66 i.** (A) L1 shed in faeces; (B) L1 matures in 5–7 days; (C) L3 (infective); (D) *Pilobolus* fungi; (E) herbage contaminated with L3s; (F) cow ingests grass contaminated with L3s; (G) L3s mature to adult worms in the pulmonary tissue.

**ii.** They facilitate the spread of lungworm larvae in pastures. Larvae located on sporangiophores are discharged several metres when the sporangiophores explode, ejecting spores.

**iii.** It can be attributed to several factors, including changes in weather patterns and cattle farm management systems, a reduction in usage of vaccine and/or common use of broad-spectrum anthelmintic treatments to control lungworm and GI parasites, which precludes adequate parasite antigen exposure, depriving the animal of subsequent immunological boosting.

**iv.** Laboratory confirmation of lungworm infection by detection of L1s in faeces is only successful in a proportion of outbreaks. This is because false-negative results can occur if the lungworm infection is still in the prepatent period. Also, disease may occur in the absence of a patent infection in adult cattle, which may have a degree of immunity. For these reasons, repeating faecal analysis and/or detection of parasite-specific serum antibodies by ELISA is recommended.

67 A captive, wild-caught, African rock python is found on post-mortem examination to have in its intestine a large nodule from which large worms are protruding (67).

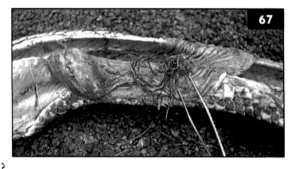

i. What is the likely composition of the nodule?
ii. Are the worms and the lesion of clinical significance?
iii. How might the python have acquired the infection?
iv. How would such infections be treated or controlled?

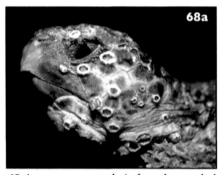

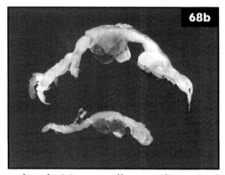

68 A young sea turtle is found stranded on a beach. Many small- to medium-sized barnacles (*Balanus* species, *Chelonibia testudinaria*, *Stomatolepas elegans* and others) are found encrusted on the plastron, the carapace, inside the oral cavity and especially on the skin (68a). Many mobile small whitish crustacea (*Caprellidae* species), about 0.5–1 cm long, are grasped in the distal area of the carapace (68b). On clinical examination, the turtle is severely depressed with mucus exuding from epidermal lesions close to the encrusted barnacles. Haematology and clinical biochemical tests reveal severe anaemia and low total protein and glucose concentrations, while CPK and BUN levels are elevated.

i. Based on the anamnesis and the laboratory results, what is your diagnosis?
ii. Are the epibiont crustacea (*Amphipoda*) found on the carapace pathogenic?
iii. What is the suggested method for removing epibionts?

67 i. Inflammatory and necrotic material associated with the presence of nematode parasites. The predominant inflammatory cells would be eosinophils and heterophils. The latter, the reptilian equivalent of mammalian neutrophils, usually contain intracytoplasmic acidophilic bodies and can be confused with eosinophils. The worms are *Ophidascaris* species, an ascarid nematode well-recognized in pythons.
ii. Their significance is not entirely clear. They are widespread in free-living pythons and it has been suggested that there is a well-adapted host–parasite relationship. When worms produce granulomata, there may be adverse effects such as blockage of the intestine, secondary infection and, possibly, predisposition to intussusception.
iii. Eggs containing L2s can remain infective for up to 7 years. The IHs are small mammals such as rodents. Eggs hatch in these hosts and the larvae migrate to the liver, lungs and subcutaneous tissues, where they moult to L3s. When the IHs are eaten by a snake, L3s migrate to the lungs, where they stay for 3 months or more. After moulting again, the larvae move up to the throat and are swallowed, moving to the oesophagus as L4s and eventually to the stomach, where they undergo a further moult and become adults.
iv. By a combination of improved hygiene (including exclusion of IHs) and treatment with anthelmintics. Killing the worms may have a negative effect if, as a result, the intestine or lesion undergoes inflammatory changes because of a foreign body reaction to dead worms.

68 i. The clinical picture, along with the presence of a heavy barnacle and crustacean load and the results of haematology and clinical biochemistry tests, suggest that this sea turtle is affected by debilitated turtle syndrome. The aetiology of this syndrome is unclear.
ii. If a turtle hosts a lot of epibiont crustacea on its carapace algal patches, they might become pathogenic. However, the main clinical sign of this syndrome is attributed to the increased burden of barnacles encrusted all over the turtle.
iii. Epibiont crustacea can easily be removed manually or by means of a brush, while barnacles require specific treatment. The barnacles should not all be removed at the same time, especially those attached to skin. These parasites are very sensitive to osmotic shock and therefore bathing sea turtles for short time intervals in fresh water on a daily basis is a good method of killing barnacles. It is easier to remove them gently from the turtle after 3–4 days of this treatment.

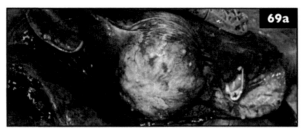

69 These parasitic cysts (**69a**) were found in the liver and lungs of a 15-year-old female Thoroughbred mare during a post-mortem examination.
i. What are these cysts?
ii. How do you confirm your diagnosis?
iii. How do horses become infected?

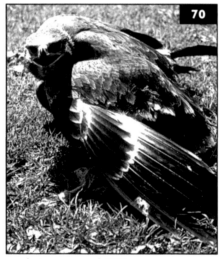

70 An injured tawny eagle is presented (**70**).
i. Which of the following groups of ectoparasites might be found on the integument of this bird – Siphonaptera, Mallophaga, Hippoboscidae, other Diptera?
ii. How would you detect such ectoparasites?
iii. Give an example of a blood parasite that can be transmitted by one of these ectoparasites.

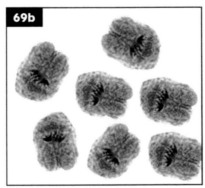

69 i. Hydatid cysts, the encysted larval stage of the intestinal carnivore (wild or domestic canids) tapeworms of the genus *Echinococcus*. Equine cystic echinococcosis can be caused by various *Echinococcus* species, but cysts from both *Echinococcus granulosus* and *Echinococcus equinus* (the 'horse strain') have been reported in the lungs and livers of horses. Cystic echinococcosis in horses is diagnosed at slaughter or post-mortem examination. The liver and lungs are the most commonly affected organs.

ii. Light microscopical examination of fluid material aspirated from within the hydatid cyst can reveal the presence of protoscolices (**69b**). Protoscolices are produced as the next generation of *Echinococcus* tapeworms and their presence in the cysts indicates that this cyst is fertile (i.e. able to establish an infection in the definitive host).

iii. Horse infection and larval development begins with ingestion of eggs that have been shed into the faeces of an infected dog/fox, the definitive host of *Echinococcus* tapeworms.

70 i. All of those listed can be parasitic on a tawny eagle. Siphonaptera (fleas) are rarely found. If found, they may have been acquired from prey animals.

ii. The bird is gently anaesthetized by enclosing it in a plastic bag and introducing a volatile anaesthetic agent such as ether, chloroform or isoflurane. The skin can then be examined with a hand lens.

iii. *Haemoproteus* species can be transmitted by louse flies (Hippoboscidae) and biting midges (Diptera: *Culicoides* species).

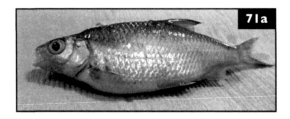

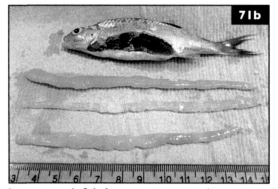

**71** A female freshwater roach fish from a private pond is presented with abnormal abdominal swelling (**71a**). The owner of the pond mentions that he has recently seen some fish with altered shapes. These worms are removed from the abdominal cavity of the fish (**71b**).
i. What are these worms, and how are they transmitted to fish?
ii. How do these worms affect fish health?
iii. How would you manage this problem?

**72** Starting with the initial infection of a chicken, describe the life cycle of the genus of parasite that causes coccidiosis.

**71 i.** Plerocercoid larvae of the tapeworm *Ligula intestinalis* (a pseudophyllidean Cestoda). They mainly affect Cyprinid freshwater fish, especially the roach. This cestode has a complex three-host life cycle with crustacean copepods as the first and planktivorous fish as the second IH. Fish-eating piscivorous birds (e.g. gulls, grey herons) act as the definitive host in which *L. intestinalis* reaches sexual maturity in a few days and releases eggs into the water.

**ii.** The larvae have considerable effect on fish health, fecundity and behaviour, and can be a major threat to natural and farmed fish populations. They cause emaciation, stunted growth, reproductive dysfunction and suppressed gametogenesis/gonad development in both sexes of their intermediate fish hosts.

**iii.** By disrupting the life cycle of the parasite and changing plans for fish movement and stocking. Control measures include culling any fish-eating birds and utilization of predators such as perch (*Perca fluviatilis*) and pike (*Esox lucius*), present in the water, to control infected roach numbers.

**72** The life cycle is split into an internal phase in the gut of the host and an external phase outside the host/in the environment (**72a** – see page 242). Chicks are infected by ingesting sporulated oocysts. This is followed by a period of massive multiplication in epithelial and sub-epithelial cells, culminating in shedding of oocysts in faeces. Once ingested and released there is/are one or more cycle(s) of asexual reproduction (schizogony) and one cycle of sexual reproduction (gametogony). Oocysts enter the GI tract and the sporozoites are released and invade the intestinal epithelia. The sporozoites develop into merozoites (first-generation schizont), which can reinfect and develop into a secondary generation of schizont. The merozoites differentiate into female macrogametes and male microgametes. These fuse to form the zygote, which develops into an oocyst that leaves the chicken gut with faeces as a non-sporulated oocyst. Further development and maturation of the oocysts (non-sporulated become sporulated) occurs outside the host. The sporulated oocyst (**72b**) contains four sporocysts, each with two sporozoites.

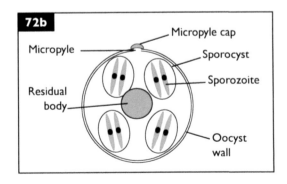

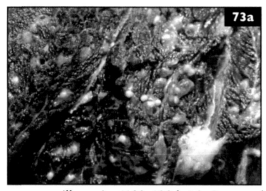

73 Groups of open-range village pigs (100–120 kg) in Peru are herded to a local butcher for slaughter and consumption. The pigs had been kept around the village for scavenging food scraps. At slaughter, numerous small cysts are noted in the tongue and in the shoulder muscles (73a).
i. Name this parasite stage and the other stage and habitat of this parasite. Describe the life cycle connecting these stages.
ii. Describe the pathological features of the muscle cyst.
iii. Describe the clinical signs that each parasite stage can cause.

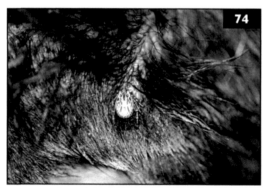

74 A concerned owner notices this tick (74) on his dog after coming back from a trip in the woods in Michigan (USA).
i. What is the name of this tick species?
ii. What diseases is this dog at high risk for?
iii. Should the dog's owner be concerned about his health, too?

73 i. *Cysticercus cellulosae*, found in pig muscle; it is the intermediate encysted stage of the tapeworm *Taenia solium*, a two-host parasite that occurs in the small intestine of humans. After ingestion of infected pork, the larvae/cysticerci evaginate and attach to the proximal part of the intestine, where they develop into 2–4-metre long adult stages of *T. solium*. The parasite can also develop an autoinfection, with the larval form of *Cysticercus* migrating

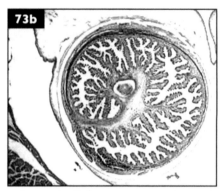

within tissues (e.g. CNS), causing neurocysticercosis. Subcutaneous cysticercosis and ocular cysticercosis have been reported. Ingestion of eggs or proglottids shed in human faeces by scavenging pigs is the most frequent way of transmission of cysticerci to swine. Larvae/oncospheres hatch from eggs in the pig intestine and migrate to muscle, liver and other organs.

ii. After 2–3 months of cysticercus development in pigs, pearl-shaped, white cysts, which have a thin fibrotic wall and an invaginated *Taenia* scolex (73b), may be seen in the muscles.

iii. In infected pigs, fever and muscle stiffness may be noted. Adult *Taenia* in humans cause few clinical signs; however, autoinfection of the CNS with the larval form of *Cysticercus* may manifest as headache, dizziness, hydrocephalus, loss of vision and nausea.

74 i. The American dog tick, *Dermacentor variabilis*, which is widely distributed east of the Rocky Mountains and also occurs on the Pacific Coast of the US. Males and females are recognized by having pale whitish or yellowish markings on the scutum or dorsal shield.

ii. In addition to tick paralysis, the risk of blood loss and the discomfort caused by tick infestation, ticks may carry a number of diseases that are readily transmitted when an infected tick feeds on the dog. These include Lyme disease, ehrlichiosis, anaplasmosis, Rocky Mountain spotted fever (RMSF) and babesiosis.

iii. The dog is the preferred host of the adult *D. variabilis*, although this tick species feeds on many large mammals, including humans. This tick species is known to transmit RMSF and tularaemia to humans. It may also induce tick paralysis by elaboration of a neurotoxin that induces rapidly progressive flaccid quadriparesis.

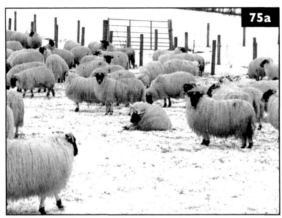

75 i. Approximately 400 ewe lambs from a flock of 1,500 Scottish Blackface ewes are routinely wintered indoors, while the rams are run with mature pregnant ewes on hilly pastures. All the sheep on the farm had been gathered and plunge dipped in an organophosphate diazinon solution during the autumn months. The shepherd calls you in mid-winter to express concern that several of the indoor ewe lambs are showing signs of pruritus (75a). Several lambs are also noted to be rubbing against the fences. What immediate advice would you offer to the shepherd?
ii. How should these ewe lambs be treated?

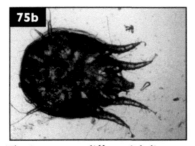
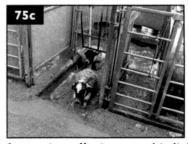

75 i. The important differential diagnoses for pruritus affecting several individuals within a group of sheep are sheep scab (*Psoroptes ovis*), chewing lice, *Chorioptes* and sheep ked (*Melophagus ovinus*) infestation. The consequences of potentially introducing sheep scab to a flock of pregnant ewes are serious, so the first concern is to ensure adequate biosecurity on the return of the ewe lambs into the fully mixed flock in spring. Confirmation of the diagnosis is important. Keds and chewing lice are visible on examination of wool partings over the body of affected animals. Sheep scab can be confirmed by microscopic examination of skin scrapings from the edges of any distinct lesions. *P. ovis* are 0.5–0.75 mm long, oval-shaped mites (75b) with three-segmented pedicels and funnel-shaped suckers. Scab-affected lambs must be treated before they are mixed with scab-free ewes. Mites can survive in the environment for up to 17 days while retaining the ability to affect new sheep, therefore make sure lambs are not moved into fields or pens that will be used by scab-free animals during this period. These constraints are not easily addressed because sheep pens may be required for clostridial disease vaccination of the pregnant ewe flock, or there may be insufficient grazing available for the lambs.

ii. Plunge dipping in diazinon or administration of endectocide injections. A single injection of doramectin or 1% moxidectin affords 17 or 28 days residual protection, respectively, while a single injection of long-acting moxidectin affords about 60 days residual protection. In this case, where the ewe lambs are to be moved to a scab-free area after treatment, there is no clear reason to use the long-acting product. In fact, while endectocide injections may be easier to perform than plunge dipping, it means having to move sheep onto scab-free pasture immediately after treatment, because of the time it takes (10 days or so) after systemic endectocide treatment before all *P. ovis* mites are killed. Therefore, sheep scab treatment options requiring immediate activity involve plunge dipping of the sheep in diazinon, taking care to ensure that every animal is immersed for 1 minute, with its head submerged twice during this period (75c).

76 You are presented with a 4-year-old male llama that has recently been imported from New York (USA) to the UK. The owners report that the animal appears 'drunk' and has been struggling to stand from a recumbent position. Neurological examination reveals that the animal is asymmetrically ataxic with the left forelimb and hindlimb equally affected, while the right side is normal. Routine haematology and biochemistry profile reveals only increased fibrinogen concentration.
i. What is the differential diagnosis for this case, and how would you attempt to distinguish the various disease possibilities?
ii. What is the life cycle of the parasite you would consider in your differential diagnosis? Are other animals on the premises at risk?

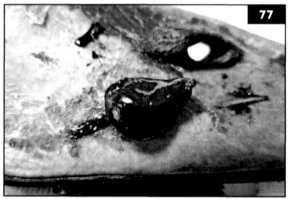

77 An adult mute swan is presented to a veterinary clinic for a pre-release health check, after previously being entangled in some discarded fishing line. During the clinical examination a parasite is removed from the nares (77).
i. What is this parasite?
ii. Is it considered significant clinically?
iii. How would you treat this swan?

**76 i.** The llama appears to have an asymmetrical lesion affecting the left cervical region of the spinal cord. Differentials include vertebral fracture, vertebral abscess, neoplasm or granuloma in the spinal canal and aberrant parasite migration (most likely the meningeal worm *Parelaphostrongylus tenuis*). Animals with fractures and, sometimes, abscesses are often in pain and unwilling to move their necks; this is not evident in this case. As this animal has been imported from the eastern USA, *P. tenuis* may be responsible for the clinical signs. Cervical radiographs will rule out a cervical vertebral fracture and myelography under anaesthesia will rule out a space-occupying lesion within the cervical spinal canal. CSF analysis may reveal an eosinophilia with aberrant parasite migration, but this is not specific to *P. tenuis*.
**ii.** White-tailed deer are the definitive host for *P. tenuis* ('meningeal worm of white-tailed deer'), but seldom show signs of infection. *P. tenuis* migrates much more extensively in the CNS of incidental hosts, often causing severe, disabling neurological disease. Adult *P. tenuis* parasites live in the subdural space of the CNS and in associated blood vessels. Adult females lay eggs in the venous vessels and L1s emerge in the pulmonary capillaries. They enter the alveoli and are coughed up and swallowed. L1s then leave the host in the mucus covering of the faeces and penetrate slugs and snails that are residing in the pasture. L1s develop into L3s in the IH. Accidental ingestion of snails containing infective L3 larvae continues the life cycle. L3 larvae leave the GI tract of the host and enter the CNS in 1–2 weeks. Larvae develop in the grey matter of the dorsal horn of the spinal cord and migrate to the subdural space approximately 5 weeks later in white-tailed deer, but persist in the grey matter in aberrant hosts, leading to clinical disease. As this llama was the only animal imported from the USA and is an aberrant host, it will not produce eggs and is not a risk to other animals in the herd. There are no white-tailed deer in the UK to transmit this disease to other llamas either.

**77 i.** The aquatic nasal leech (*Theromyzon* species), which affects ducks and other large aquatic birds. Fourteen species of leeches are described. Parasites are usually identified by direct visualization or nasal flushing.
**ii.** Nasal leeches are often asymptomatic in ducks and swans. When present in high numbers they may be associated with conjunctivitis, sinusitis, head shaking and respiratory distress.
**iii.** A single injectable dose of ivermectin (0.2 mg/kg) is usually effective for treatment. Manual removal of the leech and flushing of the nares may also be performed.

78 Over the past 2 weeks, a guinea pig breeder in the USA has noticed that 25 of his juvenile and adult guinea pigs (out of a group of approximately 600) have their heads cocked to one side or the other (78a). A few affected animals also move in circles when they walk or have difficulty maintaining their balance and fall over. Their appetites remain good, and they seem bright and alert. Most of the affected animals are young breeding stock. Necropsy of one affected guinea pig reveals moderate granulomatous and eosinophilic encephalitis in the areas of the brain consistent with the CNS clinical signs (78b). In one tissue section, a cross-section of a nematode larva is identified (78c).

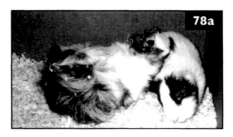

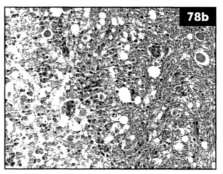

i. Localize the neuroanatomical lesion(s), based on the presenting clinical signs.
ii. What is your diagnosis?
iii. What is the life cycle of this parasite in the natural host?
iv. What are your recommendations to the producer with regard to eliminating the parasite eggs that have contaminated his guinea pig areas?
v. What are your recommendations to the owner regarding treatment of his guinea pigs?

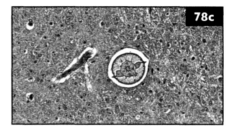

**78 i.** Head tilt suggests a lesion in the pontomedullary portion of the brainstem or the peripheral or central vestibular system. Tilt is usually toward the side of the lesion. Circling suggests a lesion in the hypothalamus or cerebrum.

**ii.** Baylisascariosis, caused by the intestinal roundworm *Baylisascaris procyonis*, which is associated with American raccoons. The breeder has recently begun feeding hay to his guinea pigs, and although the hay is stored in a 'secure' barn on the affected farm, it was purchased from a farm where the barn was not secure and raccoon faeces could have contaminated the hay before delivery to the breeder. Pelleted feed and processed bedding materials are less likely sources of contamination.

**iii.** Raccoons becomes infected by ingesting eggs containing infective larvae passed in faeces from other infected raccoons, or by ingesting larvae in the tissues of IHs such as rodents, rabbits and birds. Larvae develop into adults in the small intestine and these pass eggs into the faeces.

**iv.** *Baylisascaris* eggs are difficult to kill. Steam cleaning the facilities with boiling water is necessary to kill the eggs, but they can be washed away with water under high pressure. Bleach (or another detergent) can be added to the water to make the eggs more slippery.

**v.** Ivermectin does not readily cross the blood–CNS barrier, therefore it would be unlikely to reach effective concentrations. In some studies, the development of clinical neurological larval migrans with *B. procyonis* has been prevented by treatment with albendazole (100% protection), mebendazole (80%) or thiabendazole (80%), fed daily from days 1 to 10 after infection. Once clinical signs develop, treatment may be ineffective.

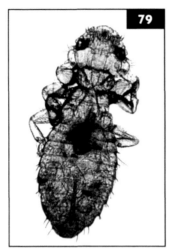

79 Canaries in a breeding flock exhibit pruritus and poor feather condition. Close inspection of the birds reveals several tiny ectoparasites attached to the feathers (79).
i. What is this parasite?
ii. What is the suggested treatment for this infestation?

80 A 5-year-old Thoroughbred gelding is presented with clinical signs of moderate to severe abdominal pain (evidence of rolling, sweating, kicking at the abdomen, flank watching). Physical examination reveals pink mucous membranes, capillary refill time of 2–3 seconds and adequate pulse quality. Heart rate is 56 beats per minute. Borborygmi are reduced in all four quadrants. Rectal examination reveals no obvious abnormalities, except for a hard, painful mass in the right caudodorsal abdomen. Nasogastric intubation recovers 4 litres of fetid fluid and peritoneocentesis recovers straw-coloured fluid with a total solids value of 20 g/l (normal <20 g/l).
i. What is your differential diagnosis for this case?
ii. What other clinical presentations have been associated with the parasitic infection included in your differential diagnosis?
iii. What is the best way to confirm the parasitological diagnosis?
iv. What is the life cycle of the parasite most likely associated with this clinical syndrome?
v. What would you recommend regarding management and prevention in this case?

**79 i.** *Menacanthus* species, a biting louse (Order Mallophaga).
**ii.** These ectoparasites spend their entire life cycle on the avian host and are easily removed by pyrethroid treatment repeated weekly 2–3 times.

**80 i.** Anything that may cause ileus in the horse. This includes EGS (UK and Europe), anterior enteritis, strangulating small intestinal lesions (e.g. epiploic foramen entrapment, pedunculated lipoma), ileal impaction and large colonic displacements (inhibit gastrocolic reflex, leading to small intestinal ileus). More nasogastric reflux is often obtained in animals with anterior enteritis and EGS. With strangulating small intestinal lesions, the horse usually has no audible borborygmi and increased total solids on peritoneocentesis. The rectal examination findings are suggestive of ileal impaction, which is often associated with moderate to severe clinical signs of abdominal pain, as is evident in this case. Ileal impactions have been associated with infection with *Anoplocephala perfoliata*, the equine tapeworm.
**ii.** Spasmodic colic, intussusceptions of the ileum, caecum and colon, poor growth and unthriftiness.
**iii.** Measurement of IgG (T) concentrations to specific *A. perfoliata* antigens using an ELISA correlates well with parasite burden. Alternatively, faecal analysis can be used, but definitive diagnosis can be challenging using conventional methods because eggs are often released intermittently in small numbers or are still within tapeworm segments. Double centrifugation and faecal flotation techniques using a concentrated sugar solution can increase the sensitivity of this technique.
**iv.** Adult tapeworms attach to the mucosa of the ileum, caecum and ileocolic junction. Proglottids (tapeworm segments containing eggs) or embryonated eggs are passed in the faeces and are ingested by free-living oribatid mites. The larval tapeworm develops in the body cavity of the mites in 2–4 months. The mites crawl onto vegetation in the spring and summer and are then ingested by grazing horses. Once ingested the adult tapeworm develops in approximately 8 weeks.
**v.** This is a disease of horses at pasture. Management is challenging as it is not possible to control the IH. Regular removal of faeces can help reduce the number of eggs or proglottids available on the pasture for ingestion by the oribatid mites. Pharmacological management includes oral administration of pyrantel (double the dose recommended for other equine parasites) or praziquantel.

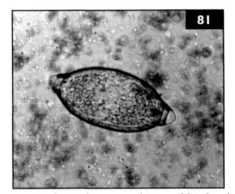

**81** During a routine parasitological survey of injured birds of prey hospitalized in a raptor centre, faecal examination reveals many brownish, thick-shelled eggs with characteristically asymmetrically opposed plugs at each end (**81**).
**i.** What is this parasite, and what is its anatomical localization in the infected bird?
**ii.** What is its pathogenicity?
**iii.** What are the implications of this finding for the avian raptor centre management?

**82** You are presented with a 5-year-old Thoroughbred brood mare that has been recently imported into the UK from a stud farm in Virginia (USA). The mare has been normal until 2 days ago when the yard manager noted that the horse was 'wobbly', particularly on the right hindlimb. Physical examination revealed some gluteal muscle atrophy evident on the right side. On neurological examination the horse appeared normal in the forelimbs, but grade II/IV ataxic in the left hindlimb and III/IV ataxic in the right hindlimb. Additional neurological signs included spasticity and poor foot placement when evaluated in a straight line. The horse nearly fell when turned in a tight circle. What is your differential diagnosis?

81 i. *Capillaria* species, a tiny roundworm that has worldwide distribution and affects a wide variety of avian species. The worms can be localized in several sites of the GI tract, depending on the avian host and the *Capillaria* species.
ii. It can be quite pathogenic, especially for some avian groups such as pigeons, psittacines, gallinaceous birds, corvids and birds of prey.
iii. The life cycle of this parasite is usually direct and fast and some *Capillaria* populations have developed a degree of tolerance to common anthelmintics and their eggs are not sensitive to common disinfectants. Therefore, reinfection of avian hosts is very frequent in outdoor aviaries. Prophylaxis is the best strategy to be used against *Capillaria* infections; colonies affected by high parasite burden should be examined on a regular basis with a faecal flotation test and the aviaries, including the ground, should be cleaned with water/steam. Flubendazole and fenbendazole are effective drugs for avian capillariosis.

82
- Cervical vertebral malformation. May have been exacerbated by trauma during travel. Usually associated with symmetrical ataxia and not with muscle atrophy and affects both the forelimbs and hindlimbs. Is a common cause of ataxia in the UK. Radiography revealed no evidence of narrowing of the spinal canal.
- EDM. Presumed to be due to vitamin E and/or selenium deficiency so is unlikely in this case as the mare lives predominantly at grass. Normally associated with symmetrical ataxia affecting the forelimbs and hindlimbs and not with muscle atrophy.
- Equine herpes virus myeloencephalopathy. Usually seen in younger horses following a history of respiratory disease and there is often more than one animal affected. Neurological signs usually progress rapidly and are associated with other clinical signs including decreased tail tone and urinary (and faecal) incontinence.
- Spinal cord abscess. Quite rare and could cause asymmetrical ataxia, but would need to be more than one to also cause muscle atrophy. Often, but not always, associated with pain and an inflammatory leucogram.
- Verminous encephalitis. Rare and although there may be asymmetrical ataxia, not usually associated with muscle atrophy. Changes will be evident on CSF analysis (e.g. pleocytosis with or without eosinophilia).
- EPM caused by the protozoan *Sarcocystis neurona*. High up on the differential list in this case because of the history of recent travel from the eastern USA, the asymmetric ataxia and muscle atrophy.

**83 i.** Assuming the diagnosis in the Thoroughbred brood mare in case **82** is EPM, how would you confirm your diagnosis? Why may this be challenging?
**ii.** Should this horse be isolated in light of the parasite's presumed life cycle?

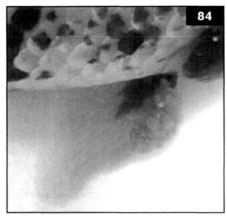

**84** An ornamental goldfish is presented with bilateral, symmetrical 'lesions' on the pectoral fins (**84**).
**i.** What are these 'lesions'?
**ii.** How would you treat this condition?

**83 i.** Appropriate history and clinical signs. Radiography ruled out cervical vertebral malformation. Other differentials can be ruled out by CSF evaluation and assessment of vitamin E and selenium concentrations. Tests to evaluate exposure to *S. neurona* include evaluating antibody concentrations in serum and CSF. The CSF must not be contaminated with blood. Antibodies can enter the CSF and therefore their presence does not necessarily mean that the horse has an active infection.

**ii.** No. The definitive host is not present in the UK and infection is not transmitted transplacentally. This parasite has an obligatory 2-host life cycle (83 – see page 243). Infective sporocysts are introduced into the food and water supply of the horse or the IH (skunks, raccoons, armadillos, domestic cats) by the definitive host (opossum). When ingested by the IH, sporozoites excyst from the sporocyst, exit the GI tract and enter the arterial endothelial cells in a multitude of organs. Meronts develop, rupture the host cells and release merozoites into the blood, which undergo a second stage of multiplication in the capillary endothelial cells, enter muscle and develop into cysts. When the muscle of IHs is ingested by opossums, the life cycle is completed by the bradyzoites within the cysts. The horse is a dead-end host, although it may occasionally act as an IH. Ultimately, *S. neurona* can invade the CNS of the infected horse only (other IHs do not develop neurological disease), causing focal or multifocal inflammation and clinical disease (EPM).

**84 i.** Nuptial tubercles. These consist of multicellular keratinous nodules and are most prominent over the opercula and leading edge of the pectoral fins of male goldfish during the breeding season.

**ii.** The condition is normal and requires no treatment.

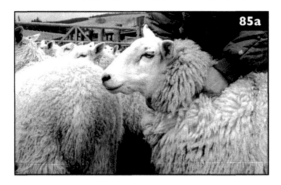

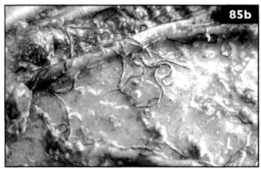

85 Severe ill thrift is reported during August in Texel-cross ewes and lambs on a farm in the east of Scotland, UK. Twelve lambs have died during the previous 2 weeks. There is no evidence of diarrhoea, but many of the ill animals are anaemic and show signs of submandibular oedema (85a). The mean faecal trichostrongyle egg counts of 10 ewes and 10 lambs were 250 and 6,100 epg, respectively. The affected sheep were all in a group of 120 ewes and about 190 lambs that had been turned onto a 23-acre field after lambing during March. The field had been resown during the previous year and had not subsequently been grazed by sheep. Another group of about 450 ewes that were grazed on 90 acres of older grass were healthy and their 700 lambs had gained about 250 g liveweight/day. The flock is closed and biosecure, with the exception of 3 or 4 rams, which are purchased annually from ram sales in the south of Scotland. All of the ewes and lambs were orally dosed with ivermectin at marking during May and thereafter the lambs were dosed with ivermectin at 4-week intervals. Post-mortem examination of a single dead lamb shows anaemia and the presence of about 28,000 *Haemonchus contortus* in the abomasum (85b).
i. Is the diagnosis of haemonchosis on this farm surprising or unusual?
ii. How might the haemonchosis problem have arisen?

85 i. Outbreaks of haemonchosis in Scottish sheep flocks are unusual compared with their southern English counterparts, partly because colder and longer typical Scottish winters do not favour survival of significant numbers of infective larvae on pasture. This outbreak was also unexpected because the affected sheep had been grazed on 'safe' pasture and had been given regular, albeit irrational, anthelmintic treatment, while the animals that were grazed on probably-contaminated pasture had achieved performance targets.

ii. Unexpected outbreaks of nematode parasitism are becoming commonplace due to combinations of parasite evolution, climate change, changing farm management practices and the emergence of anthelmintic resistance. This case demonstrates the capacity of *H. contortus* to exploit short-term changes from typical weather patterns, such as opportunities afforded by consecutive warmer and wetter autumn and spring months for egg hatching, rapid development to infective L3s and their survival on pasture. The likely source of *H. contortus* was one or more of the rams that had been purchased during the previous autumn, but not treated with an anthelmintic on arrival. The biotic potential of *H. contortus* is high enough to ensure that just one ram shedding 1,000 *H. contortus* epg could give rise to several hundred *H. contortus* in a high proportion of the ewes, which could then have overwintered as early L4s before completing their development the following spring and giving rise to significant levels of pasture contamination during the 4-week period between lambing and anthelmintic treatment of the ewes. Unseasonably warm and wet spring weather would have enabled rapid development of eggs to L3s, which might not have occurred during a 'typical' Scottish spring, giving rise to the early infection of naïve lambs. The introduction of a single infected animal might therefore result in a serious production-limiting disease within 1 year in regions where *H. contortus* is otherwise uncommon. The occurrence of haemonchosis only in the group of sheep that were grazed on previously 'safe' pasture is noteworthy and may be due to a lack of effects of *Teladorsagia circumcincta* larvae on the establishment of *H. contortus* within the abomasums of the naïve lambs.

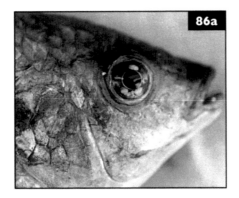

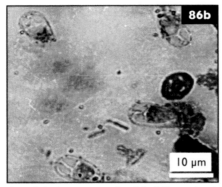

86 A freshwater tilapian fish is presented with bilateral whitish/yellowish spots in the sclerae (**86a**). There are cysts, ranging from 1–2 mm in diameter, in the episclera, causing slight exophthalmia. The detected cysts contain a large number of mature spores that have a relatively consistent morphology (**86b**).
i. What are these spores?
ii. How do fish aquire them?

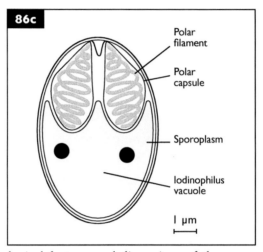

86 i. The morphological features and dimensions of the spores (approximately 10 μm long and 7 μm wide) suggest *Myxobolus dermatobia*. *M. dermatobia* was first described from the skin cysts of the Japanese eel (*Anguilla japonica*). It was reported in the stomach, intestine and gills of wild *Anguilla anguilla* in England. It was also reported from tropical countries in smears from skin, kidneys, liver and intestines of *Tilapia* species.

ii. Spores of *Myxobolus* species are composed of two shell valves that join at a sutural plan, a sporoplasm that is infective to the host and two polar filaments that lie coiled within two polar capsules (86c). When appropriate, hosts ingest the spores and the polar filaments within the polar capsule are expelled and used for anchoring. Transmission of the parasite takes place mostly through the water supply, as in other *Myxobolus* species. The aquatic oligochaete *Tubifex tubifex* (a sludge worm) (the invertebrate host for *Myxobolus cerebralis*, the causative agent of salmonid whirling disease) was found in the same location that the present fish was captured.

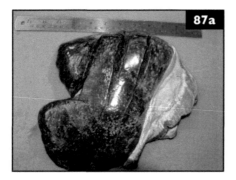

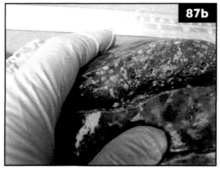

87 Ill thrift is reported in a group of sheep grazing on Machair in the west coast of Scotland, UK. Post-mortem examination of an ill ewe reveals a swollen liver with white, fibrotic lesions beneath its capsular surface (87a) and throughout its substance (87b).
i. What is the parasitological cause of the problem?
ii. How can the diagnosis be confirmed?
iii. How can the parasite be treated and controlled?

88 Why is it not unusual to see a few fleas (<10) on correctly treated pets?

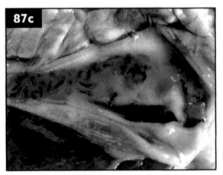
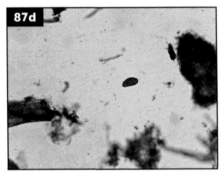

87 i. Dicrocoeliosis, caused by *Dicrocoelium dendriticum*.

ii. The 5–10-mm long, lanceolate flukes are seen in incised affected livers and within bile ducts (87c). Several thousand flukes are commonly found. Diagnosis depends on identification of *D. dendriticum* eggs (87d) in faecal sedimentation preparations. Eggs are small (~40 × 25 μm), brown, translucent and operculate, with a flattened side. The miracidium can be seen within eggs in freshly voided faeces.

iii. Most fasciolicidal anthelmintics are ineffective against *D. dendriticum* at the recommended dose rate. Netobimin is effective at 20 mg/kg (not available in the UK). Albendazole is effective at 20 mg/kg (twice the dose required to kill adult *F. hepatica*), while praziquantel is effective when given at the extremely high dose rate of 50 mg/kg. (**Note**: Praziquantel is available in the UK in combination with levamisole, and is used at a dosage of 3.5 mg/kg for control of *Monezia expansa*. Administration at the dosage required to kill *D. dendriticum* involves giving highly toxic amounts of levamisole.)

88 Because none of the flea treatments act as repellents and so the flea has to be on the pet to come into contact with the product and die. Most flea treatments aim to kill fleas within 24 hours, before they lay eggs.

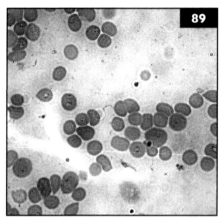

89 A 2-year-old cat is presented with depression, inappetence, a roughened hair coat, exercise intolerance, weight loss, weakness, tachycardia, tachypnoea and vomiting. A blood smear is made (89).
i. What is your diagnosis?
ii. How do cats become infected with this parasite?
iii. What public health risk is associated with this infection?

90 A veterinary clinic is presented with a 5-year-old Welsh pony gelding that lives at a private establishment along with a horse and a Shetland pony. None of the animals leaves the premises and endoparasites are managed with regular faecal removal from pasture. Over the last few days the pony has developed limb ataxia, has fallen over twice and has struggled to get up. The owner feels that the animal is getting worse. On evaluation the pony is severely ataxic and hypermetric on the left forelimb and hindlimb. Haematology reveals an eosinophilia and monocytosis and increased fibrinogen concentration. Analysis of lumbosacral CSF reveals increased cellularity, with 60% neutrophils, 20% monocytes and 10% eosinophils, few RBCs and a total protein concentration of 50 g/l.
i. Which parasites have been associated with aberrant migration into the nervous system of horses?
ii. What are the options for confirming the parasite aetiology?
iii. How can this case be managed?

**89 i.** Feline babesiosis, caused by infection by the haemoprotozoan *Babesia*. Many species of *Babesia* have been documented in cats. Diagnosis depends on demonstration of the organism within erythrocytes or positive serological testing.
**ii.** *Babesia* are tick-borne parasites. Ticks of the genera *Ixodes, Dermacentor, Rhipicephalus, Amblyomma* and *Haemophysalis* are known to infest cats and are likely vectors for transmission. Mechanical transmission via other biting insects and arthropods may also occur. Transmission via blood transfusion or vertical transmission from queen to kittens is possible. *Babesia* organisms multiply within erythrocytes of the feline host via multiple fission to produce merozoites. Ticks become infected on ingestion of parasitized cat erythrocytes. Within ticks, babesial merozoites undergo multiple fission resulting in the production of sporozoites (infective undeveloped cells) within the arthropod salivary glands. These are then passed during biting via tick saliva into the host circulation. The adult female tick is considered most important in vector transmission as transstadial and transovarial (multiplication in the ovaries and eggs perpetuating the life cycle over multiple generations) infections occur.
**iii.** The organism does not infect humans. However, cats can harbour ticks which carry other zoonotic agents into the human environment.

**90 i.** Aberrant parasite migration causing neurological signs is rare in horses. The following parasites have been confirmed at post-mortem examination as being responsible for these clinical signs: *Halicephalobus* (*Micronema*) *deletrix* – usually causes no disease in horses, but there are more case reports of this parasite than any other; *Strongylus vulgaris* and *S. equinus*, especially L4s and L5s, are involved in thrombi formation leading to asymmetric disease in the brain and, occasionally, the spinal cord; *Draschia megastoma* – usually associated with granulomatous lesions in the stomach and mild gastritis; *Setaria* species – usually cause no significant effects; *Angiostrongylus cantonensis* – aberrant migration and usually causes no disease in horses; *Hypoderma* species – horses are accidental hosts of warble fly larvae.
**ii.** Confirmation is based on history, clinical signs and ruling out all other likely causes, which include trauma, fracture, neoplasia and abscess. Protozoal and viral causes of meningoencephalitis should be considered. Post-mortem examination offers a definitive diagnosis.
**iii.** Management of this type of parasitic case is often unrewarding and options available include the administration of anti-inflammatory drugs and parasiticides (e.g. benzimidazoles).

**91** True or false?

**i.** The pathological damage associated with *Nematodirus* infection is caused by adult worms, which migrate extensively within the mucosa of the small intestine.

**ii.** Treatment of cattle grubs (*Hypoderma bovis* infestation) outside the recommended time scale is contraindicated.

**iii.** Collies are tolerant to treatment with ivermectin.

**iv.** The use of ML treatment to control *Psoroptes* scabies in cattle should not have any effect on anthelmintic efficacies against nematodes.

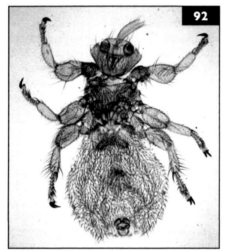

**92** This insect (**92**) was collected off the fleece of a ewe.

**i.** What is it? Describe its characteristic features.

**ii.** What is its significance?

**iii.** How would you control it?

91 i. False. Once ingested it is the larvae, not the adult worms, that cause damage by large numbers simultaneously burrowing into the gut, causing massive destruction and inflammation. A significant factor in mortality is that pathology can occur before the development of the adult stage in heavy infections (i.e. before eggs can be found in the faeces), which makes diagnosis challenging. Thus, diagnosis is difficult during the 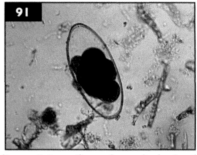 prepatent period, but during the patent period diagnosis is easily made on the basis of the characteristic eggs (91).

ii. True. Killed migrating larvae stimulate a hypersensitivity reaction, inflammation, pressure on spines and paralysis, especially in hindlimbs.

iii. False. Collies are sensitive to treatment with ivermectin because of a mutation in the multidrug resistance gene (*MDR1*) (see case 123). These dogs become intoxicated and possibly die when exposed to ivermectin.

iv. False. ML treatment against *Psoroptes* scabies could also select for resistant nematode populations and lead to reduced anthelmintic efficacies.

92 i. A sheep ked (*Melophagus ovinus*), a 4–6 mm long, wingless, hairy fly, with a short broad head, a brown thorax and a large sac-like abdomen. Legs are strong and end with stout claws. Sheep keds live on various body parts, especially the neck, shoulders and belly. The entire life cycle is spent on the host sheep.

ii. Anaemia may occur because keds pierce the skin with their mouthparts and suck blood. The piercing mouthparts cause open wounds susceptible to further bacterial and parasitic infection. Ked bites cause pruritus over much of the host's body; sheep will often bite, scratch and rub themselves, damaging the fleece. The excrement of the keds causes permanent discolouration, which can reduce the value of the wool. Heavy infestations can considerably reduce the condition of the host. Keds also transmit *Trypanosoma melophagium*, a non-pathogenic protozoan parasite found in the blood of sheep. Parasite worry and decreased appetite result in less growth and, possibly, weight loss.

iii. Dips and sprays are effective and treatment should be repeated at 24–28-day intervals. Ivermectin provides very effective control when used during routine parasite control programmes. Shearing reduces ked populations and removes many pupae and adults. Therefore, shearing before lambing and subsequent treatment of the ewes with insecticides that have a residual activity of ≥3–4 weeks to control the remaining keds can significantly reduce the possibility of lambs becoming heavily infested. The keds that emerge from the pupae are also killed.

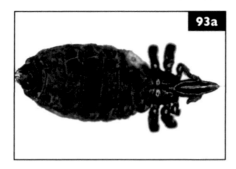

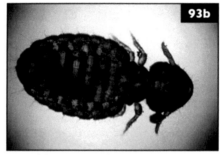

93 A debilitated, 10-year-old Simmental-cross cow is seen during April (northern hemisphere) to be covered in 2–3 mm long dark-bodied lice (93a). Several animals in a group of yearling Angus-cross cattle on a neighbouring farm are noted to spend long periods of time rubbing against fixed objects or nibbling at their flanks. Patchy areas of hair loss are seen over their bodies. Brown, 1.5–2.0 mm long lice (93b) are seen in hair partings over the necks and backs of affected cattle. Which louse species are involved at each farm?

94 You are asked to evaluate a 10-year-old Cob gelding in March (northern hemisphere). The horse is biting his distal forelimbs and stamping his feet. The feather hairs are broken. There are no abnormalities elsewhere on the coat. The horse has been getting progressively worse over the previous week and bathing the distal limbs with chlorhexidine has not improved the clinical signs.
i. What is the differential diagnosis in this case?
ii. How would you establish a definitive diagnosis?
iii. How would you manage the potential parasitic causes of this condition?

93 Lice are easily visible to the naked eye and can be picked off their host and examined microscopically. The Simmental-cross cow is infested with *Linognathus vituli* (long-nosed cattle sucking lice), which are identifiable by their long, narrow and pointed heads. *Linognathus* are differentiated from *Haematopinus* species (other sucking lice) by having no ocular points and their second and third pairs of legs are larger than the first pair and end in large claws. In contrast, *Haematopinus* species have prominent ocular points, legs of equal size and distinct sclerotized paratergal plates, which are visible on abdominal segments. The Angus-cross cattle are infested with *Bovicola bovis* chewing lice, which are identifiable by their smaller size and broad heads with biting mouthparts. Adult female lice glue their eggs to the cattle hairs (93c). Eggs hatch within 10–15 days and nymphs develop through three moults to become adults within 2–3 weeks. Long hair and a warm moist environment close to the skin surface favour louse development, hence the most severe infestations are seen in housed cattle during late winter. Transmission requires relatively close animal contact.

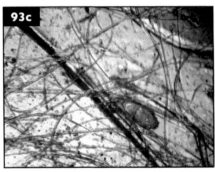

94 i. Includes the sucking louse *Haematopinus asini*, chorioptic mange, *Trombicula autumnalis*, *Dermatophilus congolensis* and *Habronema* species.

ii. Identification of lice and eggs, hair brushing, skin biopsy, sellotape preparations and identification of 'red mites' under scabs. The time of year will also guide the likely diagnosis. Lice and chorioptic mange will often be identified in the winter, *Habronema* in late spring and summer, and *D. congolensis* at wet, warm times.

iii. Oral ivermectin may be effective for chorioptic mange and, failing that, topical drugs. Management of sucking lice includes administration of oral ivermectin on 3 occasions every 2 weeks. Other precautions with lice include cleaning all tack and grooming supplies and decontaminating the stable. Some horses with habronemosis will respond to a single dose of oral ivermectin, whereas others will require multiple treatments 2–4 weeks later in conjunction with anti-inflammatories (corticosteroids, DMSO). 'Red mites' (*T. autumnalis*) can often be identified under the scabs on the distal limbs and topical insecticides are often effective for treatment.

95 i. What are the potential consequences of the infestations diagnosed in the animals described in case 93?
ii. How can the problem at each farm be treated?

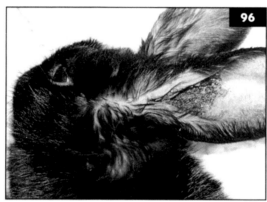

96 A 2-year-old female lop eared rabbit is presented with signs of aural discomfort, head shaking and ear rubbing of 2 weeks' duration. Physical examination reveals occlusion of the ear canals with a dry brown exudate (96).
i. What is the most likely diagnosis?
ii. What tests would you perform to establish the diagnosis?
iii. How might the disease progress if left untreated?
iv. What are the treatment options?

95 i. Heavy sucking louse infestation can result in anaemia and the presence of lice is a cause of low-grade pruritus. Chewing lice feed on skin debris from the base of hairs. Hair balls are often found on post-mortem examination within the rumens of infested calves. Animals with heavy sucking or chewing louse burdens often show ill thrift, but there is little evidence to show that louse infestation *per se* causes significant weight loss. The lice probably exploit the fact that their host is already in poor body condition. In common with most ectoparasitic infestations, the presence of lice leads to a localized allergic skin reaction, which can cause hide damage, referred to as 'cockle'. Damaged hides are only apparent after they have been tanned, so cannot readily be tracked back to the farm of origin. Therefore, the substantial cost is borne by the farming, abattoir and tanning industries. *L. vituli* has been implicated in transmission of bovine anaplasmosis and theileriosis.
ii. While there is little evidence to show any effect on production, debilitated animals will always benefit from removal of lice. Effective control requires treatment of all in-contact cattle within a period of time governed by the persistence of the product used. Organophosphate (not in UK) and ML pour-ons kill both sucking and chewing lice, but they do not eradicate them. Chewing louse resistance to pyrethroids has been documented. MLs administered as endectocide injections are effective against sucking lice, but not against chewing lice.

96 i. Infestation with the rabbit ear mite, *Psoroptes cuniculi.*
ii. Otoscopic examination followed by microscope examination of aural debris mounted in potassium hydroxide or mineral oil. Although microscopical examination is necessary to identify *Psoroptes* species, the large mites (up to 0.75 mm long) may be visible without magnification.
iii. Secondary bacterial infection is common. Rupture of the tympanic membrane can occur, leading to otitis media/interna with associated clinical signs such as head tilt. The mite can occasionally cause lesions on the body.
iv. Ivermectin (0.4 mg/kg SC every 10–14 days for 3 doses) is usually curative. Alternatively, selamectin (8–16 mg/kg topically once) or moxidectin (0.2 mg/kg SC every 10 days for 2 doses). Crusts will resolve with treatment, but may be softened by instilling mineral oil into the affected ear canals. Physical removal of crusts may prove very painful for the rabbit, even under sedation, so only the minimum amount of material should be removed. NSAIDs (carprofen [2–4 mg/kg] or meloxicam [0.3–0.6 mg/kg] SC or PO) are indicated for analgesia and to reduce inflammation. Acaricidal ear drops may be given to achieve rapid anti-inflammatory and acaricidal benefit.

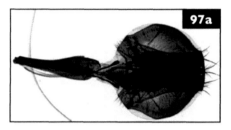

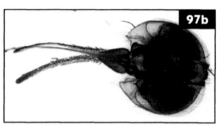

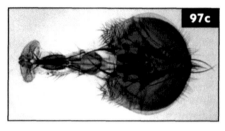

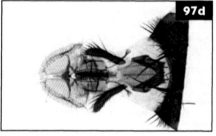

**97** Four mouthparts (**97a–d**), of four different fly species, are pictured here. What are these flies, and what is the significance of each?

**97 a.** *Stomoxys calcitrans* ('stable fly' or 'biting house fly'). It has a bayonet-like, needle-sharp proboscis which, when at rest, protrudes forward from the head. Stable fly mouthparts are relatively coarse compared with needle-sharp mosquito mouthparts. Both male and female stable flies are blood feeders, feeding on any warm-blooded animal, although horses are the preferred hosts. Stable flies are mechanical vectors of anthrax, surra and equine infectious anaemia, and the IH for *Habronema muscae*, a nematode found in the stomach of horses.
**b.** Tsetse fly (*Glossina* species), an important blood-feeding fly found in Africa. Both sexes are blood feeders. Their long, forward-directing, biting mouthparts can be easily seen when the flies are at rest. Tsetse flies serve as the IH for several species of trypanosomes that cause fatal diseases in domestic animals (nagana) and humans (African sleeping sickness).
**c.** *Calliphora* species ('blue bottle flies' or 'blow flies'). Adult blow flies do not bite because they have mouthparts for sponging only, but the larvae can be harmful and cause myiasis in some geographic regions. *Calliphora* are facultative myiasis-producing flies and have important utility in forensic entomological investigations in assessing time intervals since death. In sheep, blow flies are attracted to, and lay eggs on, fleece contaminated with faeces, urine, blood or body fluids. Although *Calliphora* maggots feed on dead tissue, they can cause considerable harm to animals (e.g. skin irritation, reduced animal growth and productivity and secondary bacterial infection). *Calliphora* have been implicated in the transmission of some taeniid tapeworms.
**d.** House fly (*Musca domestica*), which is closely associated with humans, livestock, poultry and companion animals. House flies do not bite because they have fleshy, retractable mouthparts. They are found in and around buildings and around organic wastes. House flies can feed on exposed blood, sweat, saliva, tears and other body fluids of animals. Animals respond by shaking their heads, switching their tails and becoming restless. Importantly, house flies have significant potential for transmission of diseases of both veterinary and public health implication. They can act as a vector for transmission of *Escherichia coli*, *Salmonella*, *Shigella*, *Campylobacter* and *Enterococcus* to animals and humans. They serve as IH for two horse nematodes, *Habronema muscae* and *Draschia megastoma*, which cause gastric and cutaneous habronemosis, respectively. They also act as host for the chicken tapeworm, *Choanotaenia infundibulum*.

98 It is September (northern hemisphere) and you are asked to evaluate a Thoroughbred Irish draught-cross gelding who has been stamping his feet and biting at his legs for the previous 14 days. The owner washed the limbs with chlorhexidine and administered oral ivermectin 10 days ago, which has not improved the clinical signs. On examination of the limbs the hairs are broken and in some non-traumatized areas there is evidence of papules and wheals. Some of these lesions have red centres.

i. What is the most likely diagnosis, and what are other possible diagnoses for the condition in this case?

ii. What stage of the life cycle of this parasite causes clinical disease?

iii. How would you treat this condition?

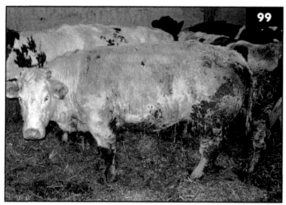

99 Several Belgium Blue cattle are suffering from severe dermatitis and pruritus (99). Psoroptic mange infestations have been reported on the farm in previous years. Despite the application of acaricide sprays on the affected animals every 3 weeks, the problem seems to escalate. How would you manage this problem?

**98 i.** Infestation with *Neotrombicula autumnalis* larvae (**98**) (the red centres of undisturbed lesions represent the trombiculid larvae). Other differentials include chorioptic mange, habronemosis and infestation with *Dermatophilus congolensis*. Although *Chorioptes* is a possible cause of the clinical signs, there should have been some improvement following administration of oral ivermectin, although there have been some reports of ivermectin resistance of this mite. It is a little late in the year for *Habronema* lesions, which are associated with the response to deposition of infective larvae by flies and are usually identified in late spring and summer. The lesions are more ulcerated rather than simple

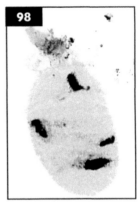

papules or wheals. *D. congolensis* usually appears initially as paintbrush lesions, which progress to moist crusts. This animal appears more pruritic than would be expected with *D. congolensis*.

**ii.** Larval stage. Adult mites are free-living and lay eggs in vegetation in a variety of areas. Larvae hatch and attach themselves to a variety of mammalian species. They inject digestive enzymes into the skin, the inflammatory response to which leads to severe pruritus. Larvae then feed on digested epithelial cells. After feeding on the hosts, larvae fall to the ground and develop into free-living nymphs and then adults.

**iii.** Avoid areas where the horse has been in contact with larvae, kill larvae using topical insecticides and manage the host's inflammatory response when severe. Short courses of oral glucocorticosteroids will reduce the inflammation and pruritus. If areas have become secondarily infected due to self-trauma, oral antimicrobials may be required.

**99** Once it is confirmed that *Psoroptes ovis* is the mite causing the skin lesions, all animals on the farm should be treated with injectable ivermectin (0.2 mg/kg). A second treatment should be given 10 days later. A herd visit and skin scrapings should be done 9 days after the 2nd treatment. All animals with acute signs and/or live mites in the scraping should be treated again as described above. A subsequent visit to the farm should be made 9 days after the second treatment and skin scrapings re-examined from animals with lesions or from animals that are treated a second time. In practice, more than one treatment is needed to ensure clinical cure. Other formulations of MLs (e.g. doramectin, moxidectin) are available for control of psoroptic mange (0.2 mg/ kg), but not in lactating dairy cattle. Treated cattle should be isolated in quarantine for 2 weeks after treatment before they are reintroduced to the healthy herd.

100 A farmer has a small flock of Suffolk sheep (two rams, 30 ewes, 43 lambs). It is June (northern hemisphere) and during the past week, three 3-month-old lambs have lost weight and appear unthrifty. One of the lambs died this morning, and one of the remaining sick lambs has brown, watery diarrhoea. The flock has been on pasture for about 6 weeks and all animals were dewormed with fenbendazole just before pasture turn-out. The lambs were also dewormed 2 weeks ago. The rams and ewes all appear healthy. Physical examination of the two sick lambs reveals pale ocular (100a) and vulvar mucous membranes. The perineum of the lamb with diarrhoea is stained with watery faeces (100b).

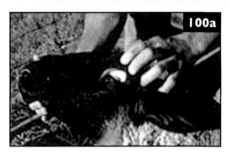

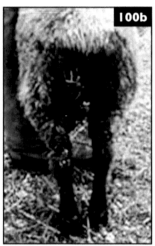

i. What parasites are eliminated with fenbendazole?
ii. What diseases or conditions should be considered in a differential diagnosis?
iii. What is the FAMACHA© system, and how is it used?

101 A 10-year-old guenon is presented with diarrhoea and abdominal pain. Characteristic barrel-shaped helminth eggs (101a) with clear, prominent bipolar plugs are detected by faecal flotation.

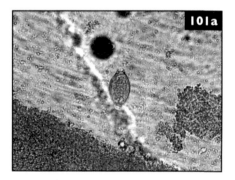

i. What helminth genus would most likely produce eggs that fit the description of those seen in the faecal specimen?
ii. What is the common name of this helminth?
iii. Describe its life cycle.
iv. How would you manage this patient?

**100 i.** Adult and larval forms of nematodes and cestodes. Fenbendazole has minimal effects on trematodes (e.g. liver flukes), has a wide margin of safety and can be used in pregnant ewes.

**ii.** Pale mucous membranes suggest anaemia associated with blood loss in an animal of this age. *Haemonchus contortus*, a nematode parasite that infects the abomasum, is associated with blood loss and, potentially, with hypoproteinaemia and emaciation/weight loss. Differentials for diarrhoea in a lamb of this age include: coccidiosis; enteric helminth parasitism (*Teladorsagia, Trichostrongylus, Cooperia, Nematodirus, Trichuris, Bunostomum, Strongyloides*); *Salmonella* species infection; *Yersinia* species infection; *Campylobacter jejuni* infection; and change in diet (animals recently turned out onto lush pasture).

**iii.** An on-farm system used for classifying animals by the degree of anaemia, based on the colour of the conjunctivae. Since anaemia is the primary effect from infection with *H. contortus*, this system is useful for making treatment decisions regarding this parasitism. Not all animals will require treatment based on this scheme, and thus the chance of development of resistance to anthelminthics is minimized.

**101 i.** *Trichuris* species. *Trichuris trichiura* is the species that infects humans and non-human primates.

**ii.** 'Whipworm', because the adult worm resembles a whip (**101b**). This nematode has a long, slender, thread-like anterior portion (whip portion) and a thicker posterior portion (whip handle). The adult male worm is smaller than the female and has a coiled tail.

**iii.** *T. trichiura* has a direct life cycle. Eggs are passed in the faeces of the definitive host (guenon in this case). After approximately 2 weeks in moist soil, eggs become mature (i.e. contain L1s), and at this time they are infective. Animal infection with *T. trichiura* is acquired by ingestion of food or water containing embryonated eggs. The shell is digested in the small intestine. Worms develop in the large intestine. They attach by inserting their slender anterior ends into the intestinal mucosal epithelium. In about 3 months the adult worm begins to lay eggs.

**iv.** Prevention of infection requires adherence to good hygiene practices and avoidance of contaminated food or water, as well as not using faeces as fertilizer. Mebendazole and albendazole are effective drugs for treatment of whipworm infection.

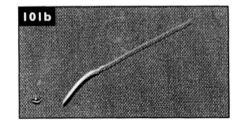

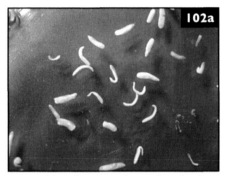

102 A necropsy on a 2-year-old male goose showed multiple small white structures within the large intestine. Low-power microscopy revealed these parasites (102a).
i. What is this parasite, and what is its significance?
ii. How did the goose become infected?
iii. What measures can be taken to prevent this infection?

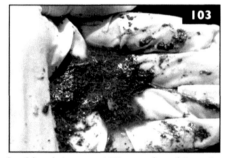

103 Necropsy of the dead lamb in case 100 reveals a thin animal with a moderately distended abdomen. The skeletal musculature is a lighter red–brown colour than normal. The blood is slightly more watery than normal. All mucous membranes are pale pink to white. There is very little mesenteric or perirenal fat, and the epicardial fat is clear and gelatinous (serous atrophy). The abomasum contains dark brown to black, granular material and numerous white to tan, thread-like, 2–4 cm long *Haemonchus contortus* (103). Intestinal contents are fluid and brown.
i. How do you interpret the necropsy findings?
ii. What types of strongyles are associated with diarrhoea in sheep?

102 i. The fluke *Notocotylus attenuatus.* Severe infection with these flukes can lead to significant losses in production. In live animals diagnosis is made by faecal examination and detection of specific eggs (**102b**). Eggs are small (~20 µm in length, 10 µm in width), ovoid, with two long filaments (200 µm) at the polar plugs, and they already contain miracidia.

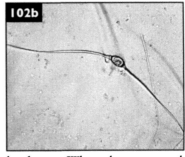

ii. Adult flukes live in the caecum of the goose and produce eggs that are passed in the faeces. When the eggs reach water, miracidia hatch and penetrate into the snail IH (*Galba pervia, Lymnaea auricularia, Lymnaea peregra*). The miracidia develop into sporocysts, rediae and cercariae. Finally, cercariae develop into metacercariae in snails or on vegetation following excretion of cercariae. Geese become infected when they ingests snails or vegetation containing metacercariae.

iii. In endemic areas, control is based on the periodic use of anthelmintics together with measures to reduce snail populations. Niclosamide, bithionol and praziquantel are known to be effective against these flukes.

103 i. *Haemonchus contortus, Teladorsagia circumcincta* and *Trichostrongylus axei* commonly infect the abomasum. Of these three, *H. contortus* is most often associated with blood loss. The dark brown to black material in the abomasal contents suggests digested blood or haemorrhage, and the paleness of the musculature and mucous membranes indicates anaemia. Serous atrophy of fat, and lack of body fat in general, indicate significant weight loss. Hypoproteinaemia associated with blood loss and emaciation is also common with *H. contortus* infection. Diarrhoea would be more likely caused by other parasites, which would make a faecal flotation examination warranted.

ii. *Trichostrongylus* species (mentioned above), *Cooperia* species and *Nematodirus* species. Their life cycles are similar and 'direct' (i.e. no IH). It is the adult worms that cause damage to the GI tract, except *Nematodirus*, where most of the pathological damage is attributed to the extensive destruction and burrowing through the mucosa of the small intestine by the migrating larvae. Diarrhoea is associated with maldigestion and malabsorption.

**104** True or false?

**i.** Lung and heart are the organs most likely to be compromised by heartworms.

**ii.** Selamectin is lethal to parasites, but it is safe for dogs, cats and other mammals.

**iii.** Because of the effectiveness of current topical medications for flea infestation in dogs and cats, it is not necessary additionally to treat the pet's environment.

**iv.** The *Ixodes ricinus* tick is known as the 'lone star tick'.

**v.** Frequent anthelmintic treatment is the single greatest risk factor for anthelmintic resistance.

**vi.** Hard ticks have only one host.

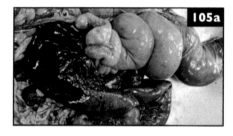

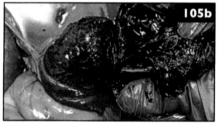

**105** A 2-year-old male Belgian Malinois is presented with vomiting and haemorrhagic diarrhoea. His condition further deteriorates resulting in pyrexia, collapse and severe dehydration. The dog is later euthanized at the owner's request. Post-mortem examination reveals an ileocolic intussusception (**105a**) with extensive necrosis, along with enteric parasitism (**105b**).

**i.** Describe the mechanisms underlying ileocolic intussusception.

**ii.** What nematode parasites may be associated with this disorder? How do you confirm the diagnosis?

**iii.** What are the treatment options for this infection?

**104 i.** True. Young adult worms are often found in the branches of the pulmonary arteries, while mature adults can be found in the main pulmonary arteries and right ventricle in heavy infection. This leads to physical obstruction of the pulmonary artery and its branches, impeding blood flow from the right side of the heart.

**ii.** True, because the glutamate-gated chloride channels activated by selamectin do not occur in mammals. Also, although selamectin can activate other chloride channels in mammals, such channels are localized to neurons in the CNS and are thus protected from selamectin by the blood–brain barrier.

**iii.** False. Because most of the flea's life cycle is spent off the host, it is important to treat the environment as well as the pet.

**iv.** False. The lone star tick is *Amblyomma americanum* and is so-called because of the white spot on the female's back.

**v.** True. Excessively frequent anthelmintic treatment will greatly diminish refugia and cause parasite populations to be under continuous selection pressure for resistance.

**vi.** False. Although some hard ticks have only one host, where the larva, nymph and adult forms develop on the same animal, some have as many as three hosts.

**105 i.** An ileocolic intussusception occurs when the ileum invaginates into the colon. Intussusceptions can occur after death (i.e. as a post-mortem artefact), but in such a case the invagination is easily reduced. An antemortem intussusception cannot be easily reduced, as the invaginated segment becomes trapped and congested and undergoes ischaemic necrosis. There is extensive haemorrhage and fibrin deposition in the lumen of the trapped segment and the receiving segment may also become congested and inflamed.

**ii.** Whipworm (*Trichuris vulpis*) infection has been suggested as one cause of ileocolic intussusception, and whipworms were found in the caecum and large intestine of this dog. Crypt necrosis suggestive of parvovirus infection was identified in the small and large intestine, plus full-thickness (mucosal and transmural) necrosis of the intussuscepted segment of bowel. Parvovirus infection is believed to be the primary aetiology, although PCR or other specific testing is necessary to confirm this diagnosis. Intussusception was probably secondary to hypermotility caused by the enteritis, although direct parasitism may also have contributed.

**iii.** Anthelmintics including fenbendazole, flubendazole, mebendazole and milbemycin. *Trichuris* can be difficult to treat and requires repeated examination and treatment. Treatment should be repeated three times at monthly intervals because of the long prepatent period.

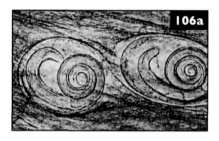

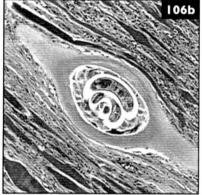

106 Members of a family raising pigs on a small rural farm develop fever, muscle weakness and oedema of the face and eyelids after eating raw pork. As part of the investigation, portions of tongue and diaphragm muscle are taken from cohort pigs and inspected for parasites. In some sections of pork muscle placed directly under a microscope, encysted larval forms are noted (**106a**). Histological sections of the muscle are then prepared (**106b**).

i. Name this nematode parasite, and describe its host range and life cycle.

ii. Discuss control measures in places where the nematode is common.

**106 i.** *Trichinella spiralis*, the muscle nematode, which parasitizes pigs, rodents and carnivorous mammals, as well as humans. After ingestion of infected muscle, digestive enzymes liberate the larvae from their cysts; these penetrate the lining of the small intestine and develop in the intestine wall into sexually mature adults, which are only 1–4 mm long. The newborn larvae are motile and reach the striated muscles by the lymphatics and blood stream. There they grow and curl up in a spiral coil within a cyst (**106a**). Larvae may persist in the muscles for a long period of time or they may die and become mineralized.

**ii.** Control is based on ensuring that pig meat is always well cooked; using microwave ovens and curing, drying, salting or smoking are not effective at killing the nematode cysts. Methods that inactivate *Trichinella* larvae include cooking to reach a core temperature of >71°C (159.8°F) for at least 1 minute. Freezing at −15°C (5°F) for 3–4 weeks can inactivate *T. spiralis* larvae in meat, but this can impose a public health risk. For example, *T. britovi* larvae (the second most common species of *Trichinella* that may affect human health) in pork can survive up to 3 weeks at −20°C (−4°F), *T. spiralis* larvae in horse meat frozen at −18°C (−0.4°F) can survive up to 4 weeks and game meat often harbours freeze-resistant species of *Trichinella*. Another approach to inactivating *Trichinella* larvae is irradiation, but this method is available only in countries where irradiation of food is permitted. Equally important is the control of infection in pigs. Pigs at highest risk for *Trichinella* infection are those raised on small holdings with minimal confinement ('backyard pigs'), because they often have access to rodents and wildlife. Control of rats on pig farms is important as they will eat carrion and be eaten themselves by farm pigs. Pigs should not be allowed to eat carrion, food scraps or other forms of meat-containing waste.

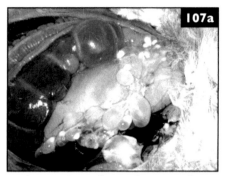

107 This post-mortem photo (107a) shows the visceral organs from a 2-year-old female rabbit.
i. Describe the lesions you see and offer an interpretation or diagnosis.
ii. How would you confirm your diagnosis?
iii. What can be done to prevent this disease in other rabbits in the herd?

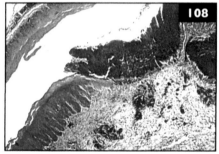

108 During the course of a zebra culling exercise in East Africa, a white-backed vulture is found dead. At post-mortem examination, insect larvae are found in its crop. Histological examination demonstrates numerous larvae (108).
i. What pathological changes are present, and to what organism are the changes attributable?
ii. What is the life cycle of these larvae?
iii. Do you think the vulture died from this infestation?
iv. Can the parasite affect humans?

107 i. There are cystic structures, which look like a bunch of grapes, on the omentum and mesentery. There is also evidence of peritonitis, with increased abdominal fluid. The liver is slightly enlarged. A diagnosis of cysticercosis is likely.

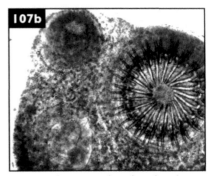

ii. The host specificity, predilection site and the structure and pattern of the cysticerci support the presumptive diagnosis of infection by *Cysticercus pisiformis* (larval stage of the dog tapeworm *Taenia pisiformis*). Within each cysticercus cyst there is a single inverted scolex that forms a stalk from the cysticercus wall. The microscopical findings of four suckers and two laps of small hooks from the scolex confirm the diagnosis (**107b**).

iii. Regular treatment of dogs using praziquantel can eliminate adult tapeworms. Nitroscanate and fenbendazole have efficacy against *Taenia*. Epsiprantel is marketed in some countries. Prevention of infection in dogs is possible by exclusion from their diet of rabbit material containing *C. pisiformis*. This is achieved by denying dogs access to abattoirs and, where possible, by proper disposal of rabbit carcasses on the farm.

108 i. These are lesions produced by *Gasterophilus* (botfly) larvae. The section shows erosion and damage to lining epithelium with haemorrhage and slight oedema in the submucosa, and infiltration by mononuclear cells and, in smaller numbers, eosinophils and heterophils. The lesions shown are far fewer in number and less in extent than those seen in the equine stomach, where each larva occupies a distinct pit produced largely by an inflammatory reaction.

ii. Adult botflies lay eggs on hairs of horses and zebra. Larvae emerge, enter the buccal cavity and eventually reach the stomach, where they attach to the gastric mucosa. The larvae remain in the stomach for several months and finally pass out through the rectum to pupate on the ground.

iii. The crop lesions, although fairly severe, are unlikely to have proved fatal. Larvae are often ingested by vultures, but in the majority of cases they do not attach to the crop wall. The vulture may have died for some other reason. There is concern about the decline of vultures in Asia and the use of diclofenac has been shown to be responsible.

iv. Humans are occasionally affected by this parasite, resulting in creeping eruption under the skin. This is caused by the first instar larvae, which usually develop no further and are fairly easily removed.

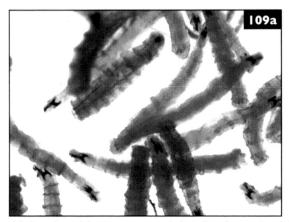

109 A 2-year-old female rabbit is presented for diarrhoea, hair loss, anorexia and weight loss. A fetid smell emanates from the perineum and tail fold region, and dermatological examination reveals traumatized skin with extensive tissue necrosis. These larvae (109a) are collected from the skin lesions and preserved in 70% ethanol for examination.

i. What is your diagnosis?
ii. How did the rabbit acquire this problem?
iii. What is the prognosis? What factors make rabbits more vulnerable to this problem?
iv. How should this rabbit be treated?
v. How could this condition be prevented?

109 i. 'Fly strike', also known as 'blowfly strike or myiasis', an infestation of skin with maggots (larvae) of certain species of Diptera flies (mainly blowfly [109b] [*Lucilia sericata*] in the UK and Europe; botfly larvae [*Cuterebra* species] in the USA).

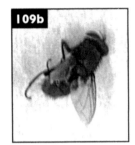

ii. Fly strike occurs when flies lay their eggs around a rabbit's anus or in skin wounds. Rabbit skin and fur contaminated with faeces and/or urine are attractive to flies and oviposition. Eggs hatch into maggots, which mature and eat away at surrounding tissues, producing varying degrees of pathology corresponding to the number of maggots and their rate of development.

iii. Favourable if a diagnosis is made early, the lesions are not advanced and the case is managed appropriately. However, due to the progressive nature of this infestation, any delay in diagnosis or treatment may result in severe pathogenic effects, multiple infestation and death. Rabbits suffering from obesity, dental problems, diarrhoea, arthritis and skin wounds are at high risk of fly strike. Flies are attracted to rabbits with dirty bottoms or wet fur. Rabbits living in dirty hutches are more susceptible, as flies like damp and smelly conditions.

iv. Intravenous fluid therapy to compensate for dehydration and fluid losses, which may be significant if large skin areas are affected. Supportive intravenous nutrition given that the rabbit may have been ill and anorexic for a number of days. Administration of analgesics and NSAIDs to eliminate the shock and pain resulting from the considerable damage to the epidermal, dermal and subdermal tissues. Removal of all L2s and L3s under anaesthesia or heavy sedation to minimize stress and discomfort. Removal of eggs and L1s, using a flea comb, to prevent the development of more L2s and L3s. Chemical treatment to kill or halt the growth of any remaining eggs and larvae (e.g. cyromazine, imidacloprid, ivermectin, permethrin). Antibiotics if there is a concomitant bacterial infection. Wound management, including debridement of necrotic tissue and hydrogel and hydrocolloid dressings to encourage wound healing. Identification and treatment of any underlying infection or problem (e.g. faecal soiling, urine scalding) that attracts flies. Advanced cases where large numbers of L2s/L3s have attacked the deeper tissues carry a poor prognosis. Euthanasia is warranted in such cases.

v. Set up fly-screens on hutches and runs to prevent flies laying their eggs on rabbits. Use insect repellents. Understand and prevent the risk factors likely to make a rabbit prone to fly strike. Regular checking and cleaning of the rabbit, removal of dirty bedding every day and disinfection of hutches weekly are recommended.

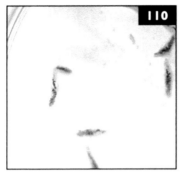

110 These parasites (110) were found in the liver of a 5-year-old Holstein cow at necropsy.
i. What type of parasite is pictured here?
ii. What are the clinical and pathological effects of these parasites?
iii. How would you control these parasites?
iv. Can these parasites infect humans?

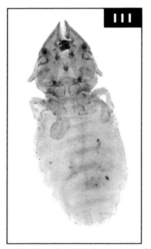

111 This parasite (111) has a distinct head, thorax and abdomen, legs adapted for grasping hairs and is found on a cat.
i. What is it? How does it live? What is its significance?
ii. Describe the life cycle of this parasite.
iii. How would you control infestation by this parasite?

110 i. The small liver fluke *Dicrocoelium dendriticum*, also known as the 'lancet fluke'. Adult flukes live in the bile ducts and gall bladder of domestic and wild grazing ruminants (cattle, buffaloes, sheep, goats, deer, camelids) and occasionally affect rabbits, pigs, dogs and horses.

ii. *Dicrocoelium* rarely cause clinical manifestations, but severe infection can lead to weight loss, anaemia, oedema and cirrhosis and economic losses attributable to reduced milk and meat production. The flukes induce chronic inflammation, fibrosis and eventual cirrhosis of the liver and thickening, distension and effacement of the bile duct. Pathological damage is attributed to mechanical irritation by the buccal stylets of the flukes.

iii. Proper husbandry practices and strategic treatment of animals. Benzimidazoles (e.g. albendazole, fenbendazole, mebendazole, thiabendazole) and pro-benzimidazoles (netobimin, thiophanate) have been used, but at higher doses than those used against other helminth infections.

iv. Although uncommon, *Dicrocoelium* infections have been reported in humans. However, the finding of *Dicrocoelium* eggs in human faecal specimens is occasionally seen as an indication of false (spurious) infection caused by ingestion of beef or other species livers containing adult flukes. Differentiation between true and false infection requires repeated stool examinations of samples from patients with a liver-free diet and, possibly, examination of duodenal or biliary fluid.

111 i. *Felicola subrostratus*, the biting louse of cats. It is the only louse species affecting cats. Predilection sites include face, back and pinnae where they feed on skin scales and secretions from skin lesions, causing non-specific lesions characterized by scaling, papules, crusts, pruritus and a dull coat. The damage to the skin from scratching may result in alopecia and crusts, inflammatory excoriation and secondary bacterial involvement.

ii. *F. subrostratus* is highly host specific and a permanent ectoparasite, with survival off host limited to 2–3 days. It has an incomplete metamorphosis and transmission occurs essentially by direct contact. Eggs are attached to the hair coat and after 10–20 days give rise to nymphal stages followed by the reproductive imago (adult). The complete life cycle may require from 4–6 weeks.

iii. The entire life cycle is spent on the host, so louse control primarily involves treating infested cats with insecticides. Biting lice on cats can be successfully treated with a single topical spot-on application of selamectin. All pets in the household should be treated. Bedding and grooming equipment from infested animals should be cleaned and disinfected. Adequate nutrition makes animals less susceptible to lice.

112 A 2-year-old female parakeet is presented with a history of anorexia, vomiting, tremors and lethargy. Post-mortem examination reveals numerous large cyst-like protozoan structures in cardiac muscles (**112a**).

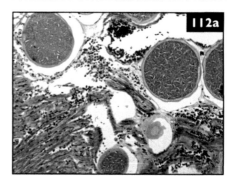

i. What are these cysts?
ii. What is their significance in relation to this bird's clinical history?
iii. What is the likely source of infection by this parasite?

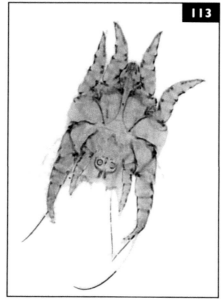

113 This parasite (**113**) is found in materials swabbed from the ears of a 2-year-old male cat.
i. Describe this parasite and its habitat. On what does it feed?
ii. What is its significance?
iii. How would you control infestation by this parasite?

**112 i.** The morphology of these cystic structures is consistent with the megaloschizont stage of *Haemoproteus* species, a protozoan of the apicomplexan group of organisms.

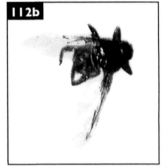

**ii.** *Haemoproteus* usually causes an inapparent or mild, acute infection. It is often regarded as non-pathogenic (perhaps because hosts may become chronic carriers after recovery from acute infection). In Europe, asymptomatic infections by *Haemoproteus* have been observed with an especially high prevalence in songbirds. However, *Haemoproteus* has emerged over the past three decades as the cause of fatal outbreaks among aviary-kept psittacine birds in Australia.

**iii.** *Haemoproteus organisms* are transmitted to birds by blood-sucking insects including mosquitoes, hippoboscid flies (**112b**) and *Culicoides* species (biting midges). The infective stage is the sporozoite, which is present in the salivary glands of the insect vector.


**113 i.** *Otodectes cynotis* (ear mite or ear canker mite) occurs worldwide in the external auditory canal of dogs, foxes, cats, ferrets and other carnivores. Occasionally, this mite has been reported in ruminants and humans. The mite is about 0.4 mm long, with a body flattened top to bottom and four pairs of long legs. The epimeres (apodemes) extending from the bases of legs 1 and 2 are joined. All developmental stages are found on the surface of the external ear canal, without being buried in the skin. The mite feeds on desquamated epithelial cells and aural exudates, but occasionally the mites pierce the skin to feed on blood, serum or lymph.

**ii.** The clinical importance of *O. cynotis* in pets is very high. Fifty percent of otitis externa cases in dogs and 85% of cases in cats are caused by *O. cynotis*. Mites are very annoying to cats. They cause severe irritation and thick, red crusts in the external ears. Eventually, infested ears droop and show a discharge. If the infestation is untreated, infection may spread from the outer to the inner ear, with possible serious bacterial involvement. The tympanic membrane may be perforated and otitis media and nervous signs (e.g. convulsions) can develop.

**iii.** Affected ears should be cleaned and an acaricide applied. Antibiotics should be given in severe cases to combat secondary bacterial infections.

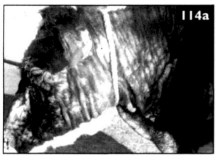
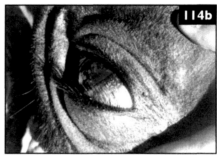

**114** From July to September, seven cows from a herd of 24 in Southern China became ill, with fever above 40°C (104°F), photophobia and subcutaneous oedema. Some cows also had erythematous udders and exhibited hypersalivation, depression and inappetence. The skin of many cows was thickened and firm, with areas of folding, cracking, hair loss and accumulation of debris (scurf) on the surface (**114a**).
i. What abnormality is shown in the scleral conjunctiva of this cow (**114b**)?
ii. What is your diagnosis?
iii. How does a cow become infected with the causative agent?
iv. How might you treat this condition?

**115** A 4-year-old female llama is presented because of a 3-day history of lethargy and ataxia involving all four limbs. Treatment with flunixin, ivermectin and fenbendazole is instituted, but the llama's condition continues to deteriorate over the next 5 days. The animal becomes recumbent and has difficulty rising, and euthanasia is elected.
i. In view of the treatment protocol selected for this animal, what is the major differential in this case?
ii. What is the life cycle of the agent that causes this disease?

114 i. There are several, conspicuous white cysts, up to 1.5 mm in size.

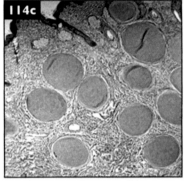

ii. The clinical signs and detection of *Besnoitia* cysts in the scleral conjunctiva or bradyzoite-containing tissue cysts (114c) in the thickened skin confirm the diagnosis as besnoitiosis. *Besnoitia besnoiti* is the causative agent in cattle. Characteristic thickening of the skin, accompanied by the changes described for this cow, is why besnoitiosis is sometimes referred to as 'elephant skin disease'.

iii. The most likely route of infection is through ingestion of sporulated oocysts from cat faeces. Other possible routes include mechanical spread by biting flies. Cattle feeding on skin lesions of other animals may be another route of transmission.

iv. There is no specific effective drug at the present time, although albendazole and robenidine hydrochloride are considered the drugs of choice for acute bovine besnoitiosis. Praziquantel is effective for chronic besnoitiosis in cattle. Suramin and antimony preparations (1%) can relieve the signs and oxytetracycline can have some therapeutic potential against *B. besnoiti*.


115 i. Ivermectin is commonly given when *Parelaphostrongylus tenuis* larval migration is suspected. White-tailed deer are the natural hosts for this parasite, but camelids are highly susceptible aberrant hosts. The parasite migrates through the CNS and can cause signs related to brain and/or spinal cord involvement.

ii. Adult worms reside in the veins and sinuses of the dura mater of the brain, where eggs are laid. Eggs travel through the bloodstream to the lungs, hatch into larvae in the alveoli and are then coughed up, swallowed, passed in the faeces and eaten by small slugs and snails. Larvae mature in 3–4 weeks in these IHs. When deer eat infected slugs and snails, larvae penetrate the stomach wall, enter nerves and travel to the spinal cord, where they mature for 20–30 days. Adult worms then move into the CSF and brain. Once in the brain, adults pass through the dura mater and into the veins and sinuses. The entire life cycle takes 82–91 days. Llamas become infected by eating slugs and snails containing *P. tenuis* larvae. These follow the same path to the spinal cord as in deer, but in the unnatural host the parasite essentially 'gets lost' and causes damage to the nervous tissue of the spinal cord and brain (instead of winding up in the dura). Infection is not contagious from one llama to another.

**116 i.** With regard to the llama in case **115**, what are the typical gross and histological lesions associated with parasitic migration through the CNS, especially in aberrant hosts?
**ii.** What is the antiparasitic spectrum of ivermectin?
**iii.** What is the antiparasitic spectrum of fenbendazole?

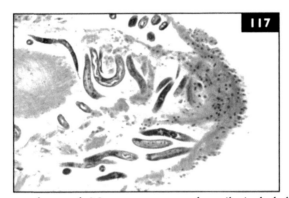

**117** Studies on endangered Moorean gastropod snails included post-mortem examination and histological investigation of all snails that died. A section of the soft tissues of one of the snails revealed these worm-like organisms (**117**).
**i.** What are these organisms?
**ii.** Is there evidence of a host response?
**iii.** What is the clinical significance of these organisms?

116 i. Gross lesions may appear as areas of discolouration associated with tissue damage (degeneration, necrosis), inflammation and/or haemorrhage. The linear or tract-like nature (116a) is characteristic of a lesion caused by migration of an adult or larval parasite. Histologically, the reaction is typically granulomatous (dominated by macrophages), with tissue debris and possibly haemorrhage. Eosinophils may be present (116b). The culprit nematode is not often found, as it will have 'moved on' in response to the host's reaction.

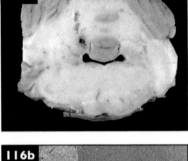

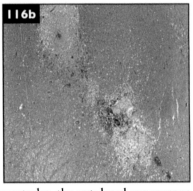

ii. Ivermectin kills nematode helminth parasites and many ectoparasites. It is not effective against trematodes or cestodes.

iii. Fenbendazole is effective against adult and larval forms of nematodes and cestodes. It has minimal effects on trematodes.

117 i. Nematode worms of uncertain identity.

ii. Although snails can be infected *in vivo* by nematodes, the autolysed appearance of some of the tissue and the absence of a cellular response in this specimen suggest that these worms invaded the snail post mortem. Free-living nematodes abound in the environment (in soil, on plants and in surface films of water) and quickly colonize a dead or dying animal.

iii. Probably none. However, the relevance of these worms in terms of captive breeding of rare species is that the detection and removal of sick or dead snails may not be as efficient as it should be. Improved management, especially regular inspection of cages, may be advisable.

**118** As part of the diagnostic work-up for an anorexic Hermann's tortoise, you perform a faecal flotation (**118**).
**i.** Name the parasite seen in the flotation.
**ii.** Is it clinically significant?
**iii.** How would you treat this animal?

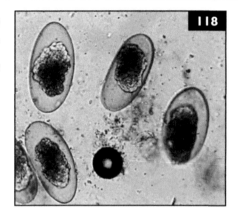

**119 i.** Match the anthelmintic drugs listed below with their mechanism of action.

| | |
|---|---|
| a. Fenbendazole | 1. GABA receptor agonist and stimulates inhibitory GABA transmission at the parasite neuromuscular junction, leading to flaccid paralysis of adult worms. |
| b. Levamisole | 2. Binds to the nematode beta-tubulin subunit, preventing its dimerization and subsequent polymerization during microtubule assembly. |
| c. Piperazine | 3. Acts as agonist at nematode nicotinic acetylcholine receptor, causing worm paralysis. |
| d. Abamectin | 4. Stimulates the permanent opening of ligand-gated chloride channels, especially glutamate-gated channels in the membrane of neurones in invertebrates, causing an ion imbalance in the nervous system, resulting in paralysis. |
| e. Emodepside | 5. Paralyses worms by attacking the receptor Hco-MPTL-1, which is only present in nematodes. This is a unique kind of acetylcholine receptor. |
| f. Monepantel | 6. A depolarizing neuromuscular blocker that has a cholinergic action on the musculature of the parasite. |
| g. Pyrantel | 7. Binds to the latrophilin receptor and the $Ca^{2+}$-activated $K^+$ ion channel (SLO-1) in the parasite, leading to paralysis and death. |

**ii.** How does resistance develop against an anthelmintic?
**iii.** What are the most common causes of anthelmintic resistance?
**iv.** Describe a protocol for monitoring anthelmintic resistance.

**118 i.** Eggs of an oxyurid nematode.

**ii.** Often asymptomatic and in moderate numbers may aid digestion. Heavy burdens may cause debility and occasionally intestinal obstruction. Oxyurids have a direct life cycle, which can lead to large increases in worm numbers, especially in small enclosures.

**iii.** Fenbendazole is effective when treatment is deemed necessary. Enclosure hygiene and prompt removal of faeces aid reduction in reinfection.

**119 i.** (a – 2); (b – 3); (c – 1); (d – 4); (e – 7); (f – 5); (g – 6).

**ii.** Worms employ different strategies to achieve a state of reduced susceptibility towards a given anthelmintic. These include: modification of the drug target (e.g. binding site) so that the drug is no longer recognized; increasing target site numbers (e.g. neuronal receptors) or amplification of target genes to overcome the drug action; modification in metabolism that expels the drug (e.g. upregulation of P-glycoprotein exporter in helminths); change in the distribution of the drug in the target parasite that prevents the drug from getting to its site of action (e.g. increased sequestration of the drug).

**iii.** Frequent treatment, treating all animals at the same time, treating when there are low levels of refugia on pasture, frequent use of larvicidal drugs, underdosing, introducing resistant worms with new addition to the herd/flock and treat-and-move strategies.

**iv.** Anthelmintic resistance should be monitored regularly. Observe and note even the smallest changes in the animal's behaviour, eating habits, faeces, coat and general condition. Perform periodic faecal examinations to monitor the efficacy of the deworming programme and assess the burden of infection. The type and frequency of deworming can be based on egg counts (testing before and after using a dewormer and looking for significant reduction in eggs). Ideally, the count should decrease by 90–100% following treatment. If it does not, this indicates there is a resistance problem.

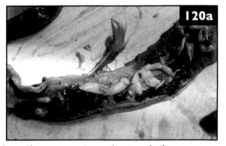

120 A 3-month-old male goose is submitted for post-mortem examination. Anorexia, emaciation, diarrhoea, anaemia and limb muscle weakness are reported by the owner at the time of submission. Necropsy reveals catarrhal and haemorrhagic enteritis associated with parasites (120a).
i. What are these parasites, and what are their distinguishing features?
ii. Describe the life cycle of this parasite.
iii. What advice would you give to the owner?

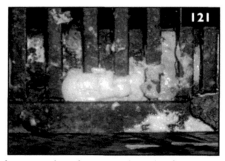

121 Several litters of neonatal piglets raised in the farrowing rooms of a modern pig farm have scours that are soft, pasty and grey (121). Most affected piglets are 10–14 days of age and have poor body condition. The mothers appear normal.
i. Describe the life cycle of the common coccidial parasite that is the likely diagnosis in these piglets.
ii. Outline the gross pathological features associated with this condition.
iii. What treatment and preventive measures are usually advised for this particular problem?

120 i. Tapeworms (*Drepanidotaenia [Hymenolepis] lanceolata*). Adults are pale yellow or white in colour and measure 6.5–9.5 cm in length (120b). The worm has a spear-shaped head or scolex bearing attachment organs (rostellar hooks and suckers), a short unsegmented neck and a chain of body segments.

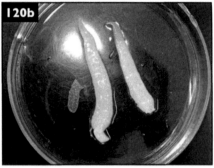

ii. Gravid tapeworm proglottids are passed in the faeces of the definitive host, in this case the goose. IHs, such as *Cyclops* and *Diaptomus* (two genera of copepods), then ingest the eggs. The embryo (larva) hatches from the egg in the intestine of the IH. In 7–13 days the larva develops into a cysticercoid and remains in the body cavity of the IH until eaten by the goose. The cysticercoid is activated by bile in the goose and attaches to the mucosa of the small intestine. Development of proglottids starts immediately. The prepatent period is about 20 days.

iii. Deworm adult geese with praziquantel at the beginning of winter and spring. Implement sound hygiene and management strategies to reduce environmental contamination and transmission of infection.

121 i. The life cycle of *Isospora suis* includes both asexual and sexual cycles within the epithelial cells of the intestines of host piglets. Numerous new-generation oocysts are passed via the faeces within 5–7 days after uptake of sporulated oocysts. These oocysts are located on the floor of the farrowing rooms for intake by piglets shortly after birth.

ii. Post-mortem examination of piglets affected with *I. suis* usually shows fibrinous enteritis, which mainly affects the middle and posterior part of the jejunum.

iii. Treatment is usually with oral or rectally delivered trimethoprim/sulpha products and electrolytes. No piglet vaccines are available. For prevention, the potent anticoccidial drug toltrazuril is recommended as a single oral dose at 3–4 days of age. The floors of farrowing rooms should be sterilized using high-pressure hot water. *I. suis* oocysts are known to be resistant to many disinfectants. However, there have been some reports of a reduction in the number of oocysts when compounds that are able to penetrate the oocyst wall are used (cresolic acid, chlorine or ammonia in a 50% solution).

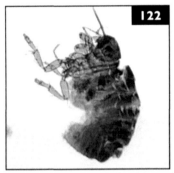

122 A helmeted guinea fowl, part of a wildlife health study in East Africa, is found to have multiple small arthropod parasites attached to the skin on its face. These are collected and mounted. One of the parasites is shown (122).
i. What is this parasite?
ii. Is it pathogenic?
iii. How might such an infestation be controlled?

123 A 10-year-old DSH cat is presented at a private clinic with generalized tremors, ataxia, disorientation, distress, dilated pupils, slowed heart rate and hypothermia 18 hours after accidental application of a spot-on ivermectin preparation by the owner.
i. If the ivermectin preparation caused the neurological signs in this cat, what would be the underlying mechanism?
ii. How would you treat this cat?
iii. What other animal species can develop ivermectin intoxication?

**122 i.** A sticktight flea (*Echidnophaga gallinacea*), one of the 'sessile' fleas that remain attached to their host rather than moving around among the hairs or feathers.

**ii.** Yes, like all fleas. It sucks blood and can make its host anaemic. Sticktight fleas cause a local inflammatory lesion and can, especially if the bird scratches itself, provide a portal of entry for bacterial infections. It may also be capable of transmitting blood parasites.

**iii.** Control of infestation can prove difficult. Hygiene is important as the fleas flourish in dirty conditions, where eggs shed by attached female fleas lie undisturbed and where the larvae can grow and metamorphose. Treatment of adult fleas is best achieved by direct application of a (safe) insecticide (e.g. pyrethrum-based product). The fleas will also die if petroleum jelly or some other oily substance is smeared over them; this blocks the flea's spiracles and prevents it from breathing.

**123 i.** Ivermectin toxicity can occur when excessive doses (not only spot-on products) are administered. The observed clinical signs are attributed to the enhancement of neuronal inhibition due to ivermectin binding to GABA-gated chloride channels that are confined to the CNS.

**ii.** The prognosis is always guarded. There is no specific antidote and therapy is mainly supportive. A propofol infusion can lead to temporary resolution of clinical signs, but these can return as the cat regains consciousness. Affected animals may remain recumbent for long periods, therefore frequent turning, appropriate bedding, physical therapy, attentive nursing care and other routine treatment measures for a recumbent animal are important. Respiratory, cardiovascular and nutritional support may be required. With adequate supportive care most animals can make a full recovery.

**iii.** The breeds of dogs most commonly affected are Collies and Collie-crosses because of a mutation in the multidrug resistance gene (*MDR1*). This gene encodes for P-glycoprotein, which restricts the entry of ivermectin into the brain by an efflux mechanism. Hence, MDR1 P-glycoprotein-lacking dogs have less tolerance for treatment with ivermectin because their blood–brain barrier becomes more permeable to ivermectin, leading to accumulation of ivermectin in the brain and severe signs of neurotoxicosis. Other breeds (e.g. Australian Shepherd Dogs, Shelties) also carry the *MDR1* mutation. Small birds such as parakeets (because of their body weight and difficulty in delivering the appropriate dose) can be overdosed with ivermectin following treatment for scaly leg mites (*Cnemidocoptes mutans*).

**124** A captive snake shows clinical signs of dyspnoea, including open-mouth breathing. Treatment with antibiotics is of no avail. The snake dies and post-mortem examination reveals parasites attached to the animal's (one) lung (**124**).

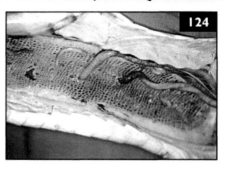

i. What are these parasites?
ii. Describe their life cycle.
iii. How might this parasitic infection have been diagnosed in the live snake?
iv. Are these parasites a danger to humans?

**125** A 2.5-year-old Doberman Pinscher is presented with severe depression, malaise, fever (40.6°C [105°F]) and tachycardia (120 bpm). Blood results are as below:

| Parameter | Value | Reference range |
|---|---|---|
| RBCs ($10^{12}$/l) | 4.17 | 5.5–8.5 |
| Hb (g/l) | 115 | 120–180 |
| HCT (l/l) | 0.4 | 0.37–0.55 |
| MCV (fl) | 60.5 | 60–77 |
| MCH (pg) | 20.8 | 19.5–24.5 |
| MCHC (g/l) | 311 | 320–360 |
| Platelets ($10^9$/l) | 210 | 200–500 |
| WBCs ($10^9$/l) | 0.3 | 6–17 |
| Segmented neutrophils ($10^9$/l) | 8.1 | 3.0–11.5 |
| Band neutrophils ($10^9$/l) | 0 | 0.0–0.3 |
| Lymphocytes ($10^9$/l) | 1.1 | 1.0–4.8 |
| Monocytes ($10^9$/l) | 1 | 0.15–1.35 |
| Eosinophils ($10^9$/l) | 0.3 | 0.10–1.25 |
| Basophils ($10^9$/l) | 0.6 | 0.0–0.2 |

i. What is your assessment of the haemogram?
ii. What is your differential diagnosis?
iii. What diagnostic test is appropriate next?

**124 i.** Pentastomes (linguatulids or 'tongue worms'). Despite their worm-like appearance, they are more related to arthropods, with an exoskeleton composed of chitin.

**ii.** Snakes are the definitive hosts, with wild rodents as IHs. Female pentastomids lay embryonated eggs in the lung of the snake. The eggs are then expectorated and swallowed before being expelled with the faeces. Eggs are eaten by IHs and larvae develop into nymphs within the host. Nymphs are released when the IH is ingested by the snake. They burrow through the intestinal wall of the snake before migrating to the respiratory tract where they develop into adult pentastomes.

**iii.** By one or more of the following: detection of eggs in faeces or pulmonary fluids; radiography or other imaging modalities; endoscopic examination of the interior of the lung using a flexible or rigid endoscope of appropriate (narrow) diameter.

**iv.** Yes. Humans can serve as accidental hosts as a result of handling infected snakes or hand to mouth contamination. Human infections are not common, but have been reported (e.g. in Central Africa where snakes are sometimes eaten). Parasites migrate through the intestine and enter mesenteric lymph nodes (MLNs), which become enlarged. Nymphs may be found in many places in addition to the MLNs (e.g. under pleura of intestinal wall and viscera [liver], mesenteries, lungs). Clinical signs of human pentastomosis may mimic appendicitis.


**125 i.** There are reduced levels of all the cells produced by bone marrow (pancyto-penia), namely RBCs (anaemia), WBCs (leukopenia), lymphocytes (lymphopenia), eosinophils (eosinopenia) and platelets (thrombocytopenia).

**ii.** Includes infectious diseases (e.g. ehrlichiosis, parvovirus infection), bone marrow necrosis (e.g. endotoxin, toxins), myelofibrosis, myelophthisis, haemophagocytic syndrome, malignant histiocytosis, hypersplenism, myelodysplasia, radiation damage, drug-associated pancytopenia (e.g. estrogen, chemotherapeutic agents, phenylbutazone, meclofenamic acid, trimethoprim/sulphadiazine, quinidine, thiacetarsamide, captopril, albendazole, cephalosporin) and idiopathic causes.

**iii.** Bone marrow aspirate and histopathological evaluation of a bone marrow core sample are required. Also, serological titres to rule out infection (e.g. tick-borne diseases, canine parvovirus infection).

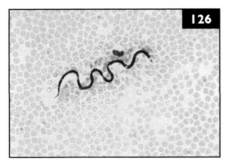

126 This organism (126) was found in a blood smear made from a dog living in a heartworm-endemic region.
i. What is it, and how would you confirm your diagnosis?
ii. How do dogs acquire this organism?
iii. Is it clinically significant?

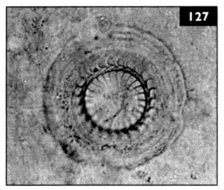

127 This organism was seen in a wet mount obtained from the skin of a fish (127).
i. What is it?
ii. Is it clinically significant?
iii. How can this fish be treated?

126 i. Microfilaria (mf) of *Dipetalonema* (*Acanthocheilonema*) *reconditum*. In dogs the most common species of filariae are *Dirofilaria immitis*, *D. repens* and *D. reconditum*. Infection can be diagnosed through morphological observation of circulating mf, detection of circulating antigens (*D. immitis* only), histochemical or immunohistochemical staining of circulating mf or through molecular approaches. *D. reconditum* mf should be differentiated from *D. immitis* (cause of heartworm disease) mf because their occurrence often overlaps in the same endemic area (see below).

| Criteria | D. reconditum | D. immitis |
|---|---|---|
| Head end | Blunt (parallel-sided) | Tapered |
| Tail | Button-hooked | Straight |
| Body | Mostly curved | Straight |
| Length | 240–292 μm (<300 μm) | 270–325 μm (often >300 μm) |
| Width | 4.7–5.8 μm | 6.7–7.3 μm |
| Acid phosphatase activity | Stains pink overall | Shows distinct red acid-phosphate positive spots at the excretory pore and anus |

ii. Adult nematodes live in the subcutaneous tissues, kidney and body cavity of dogs and other canids. Fertilized females shed larvae/mf, which migrate into the blood stream. Fleas, the brown dog tick, the dog sucking louse and the dog biting louse act as IHs for *D. reconditum*. Following ingestion of an infected blood meal by the IH, mf develop to the infective stage in about 1–2 weeks and then migrate to the head of the insect. The mf pass to the dog when the infected IH feeds on the next host.

iii. Yes, because of the close morphological similarity of *D. reconditum* mf to those of *D. immitis*, which may lead to misdiagnosis, especially in heartworm-endemic areas. Several other *Dipetalonema* species affect humans. Treatment is not normally indicated because this parasite is not usually considered pathogenic. However, the presence of adult worms may occasionally cause subcutaneous ulceration and abscessation. Control measures should be directed at control of the IHs.

127 i. *Trichodina* species, a ciliate protozoan parasite of fish.
ii. *Trichodina* infection normally results in a relatively mild disease that presents as chronic morbidity. In some cases it can cause significant losses and high mortalities, especially in young or stressed fish.
iii. Trichodinids can be eliminated by application of appropriate treatment (e.g. formalin bath, formalin immersion, copper immersion or potassium permanganate immersion).

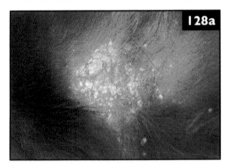

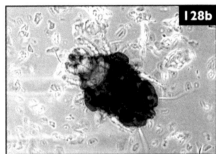

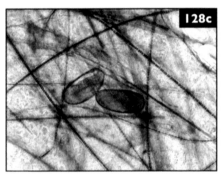

128 A 20-month-old male dwarf rabbit is presented with scaling and alopecia (128a) on the dorsal neck and shoulder region. Microscopic examination of a skin scraping from the skin lesions reveals this organism (128b) and eggs (128c).
i. What is your diagnosis?
ii. What is your differential diagnosis?
iii. What diagnostic tests would you use to reach a definitive diagnosis?
iv. How would you treat this rabbit?
v. What is the zoonotic potential here, if any?

129 A kite presents with dry, lustreless plumage. On examination of feathers, multiple raised pale structures are seen (129).
i. What might these be?
ii. How can their identity be confirmed?
iii. If of non-parasitic origin, what is their clinical significance?
iv. How might they be controlled or treated?

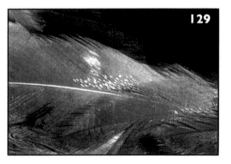

**128 i.** Infestation with the mite *Cheyletiella parasitivorax*.
**ii.** Includes: *C. parasitivorax* infestation; *Leporacarus* (*Listrophorus*) *gibbus* infestation; dermatophytosis (usually *Trichophyton mentagrophytes*, but *Microsporum canis* and other species are also reported); other parasites (*Psoroptes* mites, sucking lice [*Haemodipsus ventricosis*], fleas [*Spilopsyllus cuniculi*], trombiculids, rarely *Demodex cuniculi*, scabies, *Notoedres cati*); hair loss due to barbering (usually on the face and back of large groups of juvenile rabbits) or nest building; sebaceous adenitis rarely described, with histological changes consistent with erythema multiforme; cutaneous epitheliotropic lymphoma.
**iii.** Microscopical examination of hair plucks, adhesive clear tape preparations, superficial skin scrapes and coat brushings.
**iv.** MLs, including ivermectin (0.4 mg/kg), may be applied every 2 weeks for three doses. Selamectin (6–12 mg/kg) is effective against *Psoroptes* and *Cheyletiella*. Dusting, bathing or spraying with a cat or dog flea product (e.g. permethrin-based powder or shampoo). Selenium sulphide shampoo has been used as a weekly wash for fur mites. Do not use fipronil in rabbits. Imidacloprid is licensed for use on rabbits for cat fleas. It can be applied weekly for control of *Cheyletiella* mites. Clean the hutch and environment as for flea infestation.
**v.** While the rabbit may appear to be unaffected by the pruritus, the owner is best advised to have the infestation treated to reduce human exposure (especially young children). In-contact animals including guinea pigs should be treated.

**129 i.** Either eggs of biting lice ('nits') or keratinous deposits left on the barbs when the feathers emerge from their vascular sheaths.
**ii.** By examining them closely with a hand lens or dissecting microscope. Louse eggs will be consistent in shape and size, while debris will consist of disparate pieces of keratin. Look for lice, as the eggs were laid by them. Alternatively, retain an affected piece of feather and see if immature lice eventually emerge.
**iii.** Residual deposits of keratin on feathers are usually a sign of a moulting disorder or poor feather development, sometimes attributable to a nutritional deficiency. Full clinical examination and laboratory tests are warranted.
**iv.** Lice can be controlled by careful use of appropriate insecticides. However, small numbers may not warrant treatment; most free-living birds of prey harbour lice and only when parasite numbers increase (often a sign that the host is not preening properly) is there a need to investigate and, possibly, treat the parasites.

**130** The dog in case **125** had been treated with fenbendazole (50 mg/kg PO q12h) for lungworm infection 11 days prior to presentation. On histopathology, the bone marrow was 'hypocellular', with decreased numbers of all cell lines, as illustrated in this representative image (**130**).

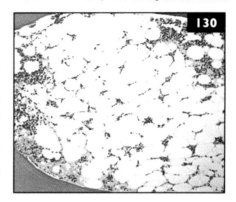

i. What is the likely cause of bone marrow hypocellularity in this dog?
ii. What is fenbendazole, and how does it work?
iii. How should this dog be managed?

**131** You are asked to evaluate a 7-year-old Thoroughbred mare used for show jumping. She shakes her head in the stable and, when exercised, rubs her ears and the top of her head at all available opportunities. Duration of signs is 5 days. The owner reports that the mare has had white, proliferative areas within the ear pinnae (**131**) for the previous 6 months and these have also been seen in other horses on the premises. As yet, no other horses appear to be displaying pruritus or head shaking.

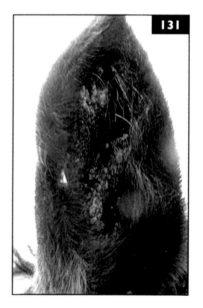

i. What is your differential diagnosis for this condition?
ii. What are the white, proliferative areas in the ears, and are they likely to be clinically significant?
iii. How would you confirm your diagnosis?
iv. How would you manage this condition?

130 i. If infectious, neoplastic, autoimmune and toxic aetiologies are ruled out, the pancytopenia may be due to bone marrow toxicosis associated with an idiosyncratic reaction to fenbendazole. In contrast to a dose-related side-effect, idiosyncratic reaction is an unpredictable drug reaction that leads to toxicity at therapeutic dosages in a small percentage of the population and has no relationship to administered dosages. The reaction may be unique to this dog in this case. Diagnosis is confirmed if resolution of clinical signs occurs after discontinuation of drug administration.

ii. A benzimidazole anthelmintic widely used in veterinary medicine to treat various parasitic infections. Benzimidazoles act by binding to parasite tubulin, inhibiting cellular division and polymerization of beta-tubulin dimers to form microtubules, thereby altering cellular metabolism. Differences in affinity between parasitic and mammalian tubulin, as well as differences in the pharmacokinetics of benzimidazoles between parasites and mammals, are responsible for the high therapeutic index for this class of drug. Despite a wide safety margin, adverse drug events associated with fenbendazole have been recorded.

iii. Withdrawal of fenbendazole, supportive therapy with fluids and/or blood transfusion and administration of antibiotics.

131 i. A foreign body reaction within the ears, otitis externa due to bacterial infection or secondary to irritants used to try and manage the aural plaques, irritation due to black flies, and *Psoroptes equi* infestation. Other causes of headshaking include trigeminal nerve neuritis, ophthalmic conditions and behavioural causes, but these usually only occur or are worse at exercise.

ii. 'Aural plaques', a condition of unknown aetiology and with no known effective treatment; it is not usually associated with irritation.

iii. Evaluation of the ear canal in horses usually requires heavy sedation or anaesthesia. History revealed that the owner had not tried to treat the plaques, the ears did not smell and culture revealed only commensal organisms. Cytology from the discharge within the ear and inner pinna scraping revealed a 6-legged mite larva with an oval-shaped body consistent with *Psoroptes equi*. This condition is reportable in the USA (but not in the UK), as it is highly contagious to other horses.

iv. All tack and other potential fomites need thorough washing. Administration of oral ivermectin every 2 weeks for 2–3 treatments should be effective at treating this parasite. Topical fipronil and other products have also been used.

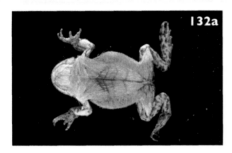

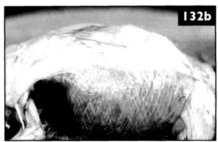

132 A toad is observed by a keen naturalist to be lethargic. It is easily caught and examined. Post-mortem examination reveals a streaked appearance to the body musculature (132a). A closer view (132b) illustrates these lesions better. A histological section (132c) shows the remains of a parasitic organism.

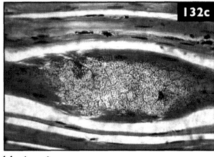

i. Which species of toad is this?
ii. What are the features of the histological lesions?
iii. What are the reservoir hosts of the causal organism?

133 You are asked to evaluate a 17-month-old unbroken Cob filly that has been coughing for approximately 4 weeks. The filly lives with three adult horses and two donkeys. The filly has an increased respiratory rate. She is treated with an appropriate dose of oral clenbuterol administered twice daily in feed for 4 weeks, but there is no improvement. At the end of the treatment period, tracheal wash cytology reveals increased cellularity due in part to a slightly increased non-degenerate neutrophil population (40%; normal range <30%), but mainly because of an increased eosinophil population (25%; normal range <5%). None of the other horses on the farm are showing clinical signs of illness.
i. What is the most likely cause of these findings?
ii. How would you confirm your diagnosis?
iii. What other samples would you obtain from the other equids to evaluate if they are affected?
iv. How would you treat this condition?

**132 i.** Common toad (*Bufo bufo*), a typical bufonid species.

**ii.** This is a naturally occurring case of plistophorosis, an infection with the parasite *Plistophora myotrophica*, which is a microsporidian protozoan parasite (Myxosporidia) of toads. Affected amphibians become emaciated and die. The striated muscles of the body wall and limbs contain depots of fusiform organisms, giving an appearance of white lines (**132b**). These parasites are clearly visible when sections are stained with Giemsa and Feulgen (**132c**).

**iii.** Fish and invertebrates. The life cycle of the parasite is uncertain.

**133 i.** This horse may be suffering from inflammatory airway disease, but the increased percentage of eosinophils on cytology is suggestive of a parasitic infection. This could be due to pulmonary migration of *Parascaris equorum*, but because the filly lives with two donkeys, *Dictyocaulus arnfieldi* is a possibility. *D. arnfieldi* is a patent infection in donkeys, but rarely causes clinical signs. However, this lungworm may cause clinical signs in horses, but the parasites rarely develop into adults (become patent). Bacterial pneumonia can occur as a primary disease or be secondary to parasitic infections, but the neutrophil percentage would usually be higher if bacteria were involved and the neutrophils would appear degenerate on cytology.

**ii.** As this disease rarely reaches patency in the horse, eggs are rarely if ever found in horses' faeces. However, it may be possible to identify *D. arnfieldi* larvae on cytological evaluation, either within the mucus in tracheal wash samples or in bronchoalveolar lavage fluid. Eosinophilia is sometimes identified on haematological evaluation. Definitive diagnosis can be problematic and evaluation of in-contacts may be required.

**iii.** As the disease is often patent in donkeys, larvae or adults may be identified on transbronchial endoscopic examination or visualized on cytological evaluation of tracheal or bronchoalveolar washes. The Baermann technique can be used to confirm the presence of larvae in faeces when the infection is patent.

**iv.** Treat the affected horse and in-contact animals, particularly the donkeys, with ivermectin or moxidectin. Occasionally, an inflammatory response to the dying larvae (and occasionally adults) develops within the lungs and requires treatment with oral glucocorticosteroids. Sometimes, a concurrent secondary bacterial infection is present and requires treatment with systemic or inhaled antimicrobial agents.

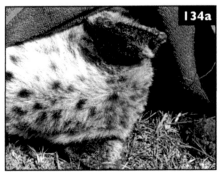

**134** The ear of a 7-year-old female wild cheetah is shown (**134a**). Note the lichenification and scaling. There are also skin lesions on the neck and various sites of the head.
**i.** What is this cheetah's dermatological problem?
**ii.** What diagnostic test is most cost-effective in making a definitive diagnosis?
**iii.** How did the cheetah most likely contract this condition?
**iv.** How should she be treated?

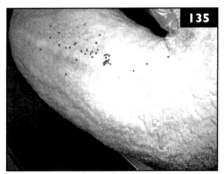

**135** Ticks are significant ectoparasites, infesting almost all animal species. Ticks infesting a sheep are shown (**135**). Not only do ticks cause direct damage, but they are also important vectors of a number of infections. How can tick infestation be controlled?

134 i. Dermatitis due to itching and scratching of the skin. Mange caused by *Sarcoptic scabiei* has been found in cheetahs as young as 6 months old. However, it is common in adults 7–9 years old and tends to be severe in older cheetahs.

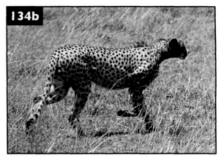

ii. Microscopical examination of skin scrapes for detection of the mites and eggs.
iii. In the wild, cheetahs are more likely to become infested with *S. scabiei* via contact with one of its infested prey hosts. Thomson's gazelles are select prey for cheetahs. They are commonly infested, therefore may act as a reservoir to maintain the life cycle in the wild.
iv. The cheetah should be immobilized before treatment (1.6 mg of medetomidine plus 1.6 mg of ketamine). Ivermectin (0.2 mg/kg) should be administered subcutaneously three times with 7-day intervals. Mange can cause skin itching, leading to abrasions, scratching and ulceration, which may cause death as a result of secondary bacterial infection and septicaemia. Penicillin/amoxicillin-based antibiotics should be given as well. Iodine may be applied topically on the resultant scab (134b).

135 Many chemical products are useful against ticks including, but not limited to:
• Phenylpyrazol. High safety margin in dogs as well as cats due to a selective action on invertebrate GABA receptors.
• Formamidine. Has a selective action on octopamine receptors. Amitraz, a formamidine acaricide, is one of the most popular acaricides for the control of cattle ticks *Rhipicephalus* (*Boophilus*) *microplus*.
• Pyrethroids. Long-term effect varies (from some days to several weeks) according to pharmaceutical forms.
• Organophosphates (licensed products not available in the UK). Have no long-term effect and are used more for treatment rather than prevention. Acaricides are usually applied by dipping, spraying, spot-on, pour-on or slow-release ear tags.

Organophosphates, pyrethroids and MLs have all been employed. Some acaricides prevent infestation for a number of weeks following treatment. Organophosphate dips give about 3–6 weeks' protection and kill all ectoparasites residing on the animal. However, concerns about exposure to and disposal of large volumes of toxic chemicals are leading farmers increasingly to select pour-on treatments in preference to dips.

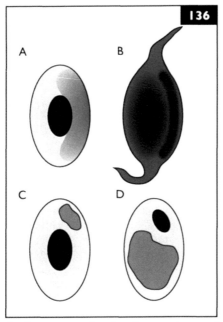

**136** During a survey for haemoparasites in a large avian zoological collection, you find several suspected extracellular and intracellular organisms in leucocytes or RBCs (**136A–D**, Wright's-stained peripheral blood smears).
i. Identify the parasites, and name their IHs/vectors.
ii. What are the clinical signs associated with these parasites?
iii. How would you control these parasites?

**137** Given the rise of acaricide resistance and the decreasing rate of discovery of new antiparasitics, using alternative non-chemical approaches for tick control is essential. Discuss some of these non-conventional approaches.

**136 i.** (A) *Haemoproteus* species (louse flies [Hippoboscidae], biting midges [*Culicoides*]); (B) *Leucocytozoon* species (black flies [Simuliidae] and *Culicoides*); (C, D) *Plasmodium* species (mosquitoes).

**ii.** *Haemoproteus* species are usually considered non-pathogenic and clinical signs (e.g. anaemia) are rare; some species of *Leucocytozoon* species are pathogenic and the most frequent clinical signs are anaemia, dyspnoea, spleno/hepatomegaly and occasionally death; for *Plasmodium* species there are non-pathogenic, pathogenic and highly pathogenic strains that may cause anaemia, anorexia, depression, dyspnoea and death.

**iii.** Prevent exposure of birds to the IHs/vectors.

**137** Non-conventional approaches include:

- Agronomical measures. Destroy tick areas by restricting animals to low-ground, tick-free pastures and keeping grass and weeds cut short in tick-infested areas. Lowering the stocking rate of animals has also been shown to lower tick populations, as it is more difficult for questing ticks to find a host. Establishment of tick-free areas is hampered by the presence of small wild mammals, which harbour and transport the immature stages of multiple-host tick species, acting as reservoirs of infection.
- Biological control. Use of tick predators such as oxpecker birds and entomopathogenic fungi (e.g. *Metarhizium anisopliae*, *Beauveria bassiana*).
- Pheromone-based technologies. Anti-tick products based on these technologies can be exploited to aid tick control.
- Tick resistant animals. Genetically resistant animals that show a heritable ability to be resistant to tick infestation can be an important element of many tick control strategies (e.g. the one-host cattle tick *Rhipicephalus* [*Boophilus*] *microplus*).
- Vaccination. The vaccine against the cattle tick *R. microplus* is the only commercial tick vaccine available, and only in Australia and Cuba.

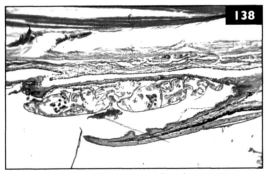

**138** A captive garter snake is found dead at a local zoo. On post-mortem examination it is found to have pale muscles and viscera and occasional petechial haemorrhages. Heart blood culture yields a pure culture of the bacterium *Aeromonas hydrophila*. Closer examination of the skin of the snake's ventral surfaces reveals small dark particles between the scales, apparently adherent to the underlying tissues. A histological section is prepared (**138**).
**i.** What does this reveal?
**ii.** Is there any zoonotic implication?
**iii.** What advice would you provide to staff and visitors?

**139** A 2-year-old male cat is presented with tachypnoea, dyspnoea, increased breathing sounds and coughing. Heartworm disease is suspected because the cat came from a region where heartworm infection is common in dogs.
**i.** What other signs would you expect to see if the cat has heartworm disease?
**ii.** Why is diagnosis of heartworm disease in cats challenging?
**iii.** How would you treat a cat with heartworm?

**138 i.** A mite, probably the snake mite *Ophionyssus natricis*, between two scales.
**ii.** *O. natricis* can cause skin lesions in some people either directly or through a hypersensitivity reaction to the mite or its exoskeleton.
**iii.** Health and safety regulations usually require that a proper risk assessment is carried out before staff or visitors at a facility with reptiles handle them, as they may harbour mites such as *O. natricis*. Even shed reptilian skins may contain mites or mite remains.

**139 i.** A right-sided heart murmur if worms disrupt the tricuspid valve. GI signs such as vomiting can be seen. Rarely, syncope, neurological signs, embolic events and caval syndrome are reported. Clinical signs are most likely to manifest in cats during initial worm migration into the pulmonary arteries or at the time of death of the worms. Cats tend to have more lung damage than dogs, because worms die faster in cats. Sudden death occurs due to acute respiratory failure from pulmonary thromboembolism.
**ii.** False negatives are common in cats due to the low worm burdens, light antigen load, all-male infection and the fact that cats are rarely microfilaraemic (i.e. blood evaluation for larvae is very insensitive). Therefore, a thorough diagnostic approach using a combination of chest radiographs, serology (for both antibody and antigen) and echocardiography is necessary. Necropsy confirmation of heartworm disease is the 'gold standard'.
**iii.** Treatment is difficult in cats because sudden worm death caused by treatment with adulticides can lead to severe inflammatory reaction and thromboembolic complications. Cats with mild signs may resolve the infection on their own. Oxygen, bronchodilators (e.g. theophylline), corticosteroids and/or IV fluids are considered a standard medical treatment in cats with severe signs. Microfilaricide treatment is usually unnecessary since cats have few circulating microfilariae. Surgical treatment, where adult worms are physically removed from the heart, is indicated in cats that develop vena cava syndrome.

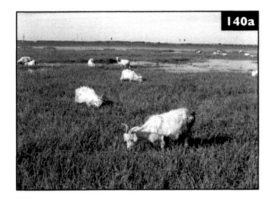

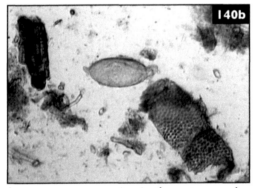

140 A flock of cashmere goats are grazing in the water meadows in Heilongjiang Province, China (140a). Four months later, all the animals exhibit diarrhoea, anaemia, emaciation, jaundice and abdominal distension. Examination of faecal samples from some of the goats reveals parasite eggs with a terminal spine and a short appendage at the other end (140b).

i. What is this parasite?
ii. Could this be the causal agent of the clinical signs?
iii. How do goats become infected with this parasite?
iv. How would you treat the affected goats?
v. What measures would you take to prevent this infection?

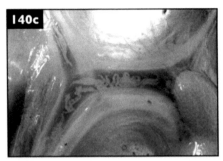

**140 i.** *Orientobilharzia* species, a blood fluke that causes orientobilharziosis in cashmere goats and other farm animals.

**ii.** Yes. During the acute phase of the disease, severe ascites is seen and numerous male–female fluke pairs can be found in the mesenteric veins on necropsy (**140c**). However, other factors may be involved in the signs, therefore it is important to perform haematological and serum biochemistry analyses on the diseased goats to rule out other infections.

**iii.** Adult blood flukes are parasites of veins of the digestive tracts of animals. Sexes are separate and the slender female resides in the gynecophoric canal of the stouter male. Females produce eggs that are excreted in the host's faeces. These hatch in water and the miracidia penetrate appropriate snails (e.g. *Radix auricularia*), where they undergo several developmental stages (mother sporocysts, daughter sporocysts, cercariae). Cercariae escape from the snail and have a short free-swimming life in water. When they come into contact with the final host (goats), cercariae penetrate directly through the skin, losing their tails in the process, and invade the circulatory system. The schistosomula or young flukes travel via the blood stream through the heart and lungs to the portal and mesenteric veins and develop into adults.

**iv.** Praziquantel (30 mg/kg) is the drug of choice against both immature and adult blood flukes in sheep and goats. To avoid the toxicosis caused by large numbers of dead worms, in severe cases the dose should be reduced to 15 mg/kg for initial treatment and repeated after 2 days.

**v.** Avoid grazing water meadows, provide a piped water supply to troughs and prevent access to natural water. Regular application of a molluscicide at the water source and manual removal of snails may be necessary. Prophylactic deworming of animals in endemic areas is recommended. Warn the owners that this disease has zoonotic potential.

**141** True or false?
**i.** Dogs undergoing adulticide therapy for heartworm disease must be hospitalized.
**ii.** Adult *Trichuris vulpis* (whipworms) live in the small intestine of the dog.
**iii.** A single treatment is often enough to treat an animal infested with mites.
**iv.** Ivermectin should not be given to a heartworm-infected dog until the dog is tested negative for the presence of microfilariae.
**v.** Controlling soft tick infestation is difficult.
**vi.** Ticks are insects.

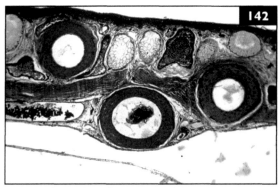

**142** A colony of clawed toads is found to exhibit skin lesions. A biopsy, taken under anaesthesia, reveals these parasites (**142**).
**i.** Describe the environment in which clawed toads live in the wild.
**ii.** What might be the relevance of such an environment to the spread of microbial organisms?
**iii.** What does the biopsy show?
**iv.** Name the parasite.

**141 i.** True, because severe post-treatment cardio-pulmonary complications sometimes occur.

**ii.** False. Whipworms normally live in the large intestine.

**iii.** False. Repeated treatment is necessary to kill newly emerged larvae and nymphs. Some products have long-lasting activity (e.g. MLs on cattle, some on sheep, organophosphate dips for sheep).

**iv.** True, because ivermectin may induce a hyper-sensitivity reaction in microfilariae-positive animals.

**v.** True, because soft ticks do not live on the host; they feed and then retire to the environment, where they can survive for extended periods.

**vi.** False, because ticks are arachnids and possess four pairs of legs (**141a**). Insects have only three pairs of legs and their bodies are composed of head, thorax and abdomen (**141b**). Larval ticks also possess four pairs of legs.

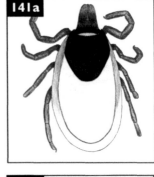

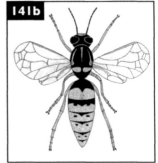

**142 i.** They are almost entirely aquatic, living in ponds, wells and drains.

**ii.** The spread of parasites and 'microparasites' such as bacteria is facilitated if the volume of water is small and hygiene is poor.

**iii.** Neuromasts of the affected toad, which have become dark in colour as a result of proliferation of melanophores.

**iv.** The metacercariae causing this syndrome are strigeid trematodes (genus *Neasus*). These digenetic flukes usually occur in an encysted or non-encysted larval form in the tissues of aquatic animals, especially amphibians such as clawed toads. The adult worms develop to sexual maturity in the intestine of birds (final host), where they can cause tissue reactions including enteritis.

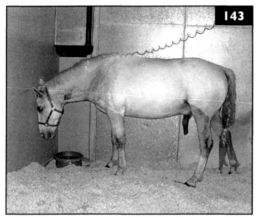

143 A 5-year-old gelding, purchased 12 months ago, presented with loose faeces, depression, dark pink mucous membranes and poor pulse quality (143). Rectal examination revealed very loose faeces and ~2-cm long larvae were present on the rectal glove. Peritoneocentesis recovered straw-coloured fluid with total solids of 25 g/l (normally <20g/l). The horse had been dewormed in the 8 months since purchase with oral pyrantel administered every 6 weeks. It was also treated with praziquantel 4 months ago.

i. What parasite larvae do you think were present on the rectal glove?

ii. If your diagnosis is correct, how would you manage this case?

# 143: Answer

**143 i.** Cyathostomins (also known as small redworms), the most prevalent and pathogenic parasites of horses today.
**ii.** This horse has severe hypovolaemia due to fluid sequestration into the GI tract secondary to the inflammatory response in the colonic wall. Management involves eradication of the L4s, control of the inflammatory response and correction of the hypovolaemia. The most effective treatments for killing L4s are a 5-day course of fenbendazole and a single dose of moxidectin. In animals with clinical disease, the burden of hypobiotic larvae is large and it is possible to worsen the clinical signs by triggering a more marked inflammatory response to the dying larvae. Therefore, pre-treating with dexamethasone is necessary prior to administration of the anthelmintic. This will dampen the inflammatory response to the emerging larvae. It is then necessary to manage the hypovolaemia, colitis and peritonitis. This involves administration of IV fluids, other anti-inflammatories (e.g. flunixin meglumine) and antimicrobials to prevent secondary bacterial infection or if bacteraemia is suspected. Bismuth subsalicylate or codeine is not beneficial in these cases. However, the former is reported to have topical anti-inflammatory properties and may be used in certain cases. Care must be taken when administering codeine as secondary bacterial infections have been associated with larval cyathostomosis; it is usually reserved for management of chronic cases. This horse may be at risk of developing laminitis so prophylactic support in the form of cooling the feet with ice and foot pads may be recommended. Acetylpromazine is contraindicated as the drug would further reduce perfusion to the GI tract and may predispose the horse to collapse. The horse's appetite is likely to be reduced so it should be offered tasty feeds, and triglyceride concentrations should be monitored.

**144 i.** What aspect of the life cycle of the parasite described in case **143** allows it to be so successful and a common cause of diarrhoeal disease in horses in the 21st century?
**ii.** Why has this animal developed parasitic disease despite the use of a deworming protocol?

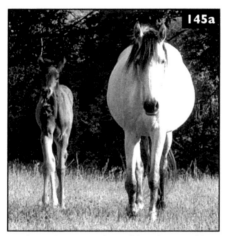

**145** You are presented with a 10-day-old Thoroughbred filly with mild to moderate diarrhoea. The foal is otherwise bright, alert and responsive and has normal parameters on clinical examination (**145a**). The dam is normal.
**i.** What is your differential diagnosis for this case?
**ii.** How would you confirm your most likely parasite-related diagnosis?
**iii.** Which drugs would be most effective for treatment of this condition?

**144 i.** Its success relates to its hypobiotic phase where L3s enter the colonic wall and are largely non-susceptible to anthelmintics. Resistance in adults and susceptible late-stage larvae has been reported for all classes of anthelmintics, particularly the benzimidazoles. As this is a prepatent disease, using a worm egg count to assess the degree of infection and hypobiotic worm burden is not accurate and does not predict the likelihood of developing clinical disease.

**ii.** Most likely because the horse had not received an adequate deworming protocol prior to purchase and the larvae were in their hypobiotic phase (in refugia) and thus were not susceptible to the anthelmintics administered. Another reason is that the cyathostomin population was partly or largely resistant to the anthelmintics administered prior to purchase and since.

**145 i.** 'Foal heat' diarrhoea is of unknown cause, but may relate to changes in diet and diet composition or may be due to changes in GI structure and function at this age. Diarrhoea may also be associated with infectious agents (e.g. *Cryptosporidium*, rotavirus, bacteria [*Escherichia coli*, *Clostridium perfringens*, *C. difficile*]). *Strongyloides westeri* (threadworms) is a possible parasitic causative agent.

**ii.** By evaluating faeces for the characteristic eggs produced by *S. westeri* (**145b**). As the prepatent period is 5–7 days, eggs may not be evident in the faeces. Response to anthelmintic therapy can also be used in these cases as a diagnostic tool, but foal heat diarrhoea will resolve spontaneously.

**iii.** Benzimidazole or ivermectin anthelmintics (many not licensed in the UK for foals this young). Ivermectin and thiabendazole can be used in the USA.

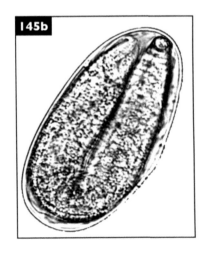

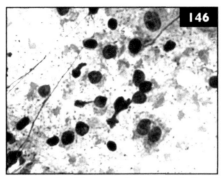

146 The body of a 5-month-old spayed female Labrador Retriever, which presumably died of canine distemper (clinical signs included depression, inappetence, hypermetria, ataxia, blindness and circling), is submitted for post-mortem evaluation. A cytological imprint preparation of the brain is made (146).
i. What does this smear reveal?
ii. What further diagnostic tests are indicated to confirm the diagnosis?
iii. How can this disease be treated in a live dog?
iv. Is there zoonotic potential?

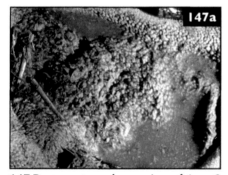
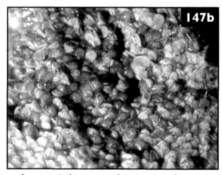

147 Post-mortem observation of 4- to 8-mm long, pink, conical parasites between the papillae on the ventral wall of the rumen (147a, b) and along the margins of the reticular groove of both sheep and cattle has become commonplace throughout the UK and Ireland.
i. What are these parasites?
ii. What is their clinical significance?

**146 i.** The obligate intracellular microsporidial parasite *Encephalitozoon cuniculi*, the agent of canine encephalitozoonosis. *E. cuniculi* has been occasionally identified as a cause of neurological or renal disease in dogs, with fatal consequences in puppies. The main clinical manifestation of canine encephalitozoonosis is an encephalitis–nephritis syndrome, which can be confused with canine distemper. *E. cuniculi* is best known as a cause of subclinical granulomatous encephalitis and nephritis in rabbits and rodents.
**ii.** Parasite spores can be detected in faeces and/or urinary sediments from infected dogs. Other tests include *in-vitro* culture of parasites from fresh brain and/or kidney tissues and serological detection of anti-parasite antibodies. Definitive identification of *Encephalitozoon* is achieved by ultrastructural examination, whereas species and strain identification is dependent on DNA analysis using PCR.
**iii.** No treatment has been reported for use in dogs. Albendazole (a benzimidazole), is not approved for use in dogs, but it might be an off-label treatment option.
**iv.** Human infection, via ingestion or inhalation of infective *E. cuniculi* spores, has been reported, particularly in immunocompromised patients.

**147 i.** *Paramphistomum* species, trematode parasites with a worldwide distribution (in the UK and Ireland, *Paramphistomum cervi* is the most likely species). They have a two-host life cycle involving ruminants as final hosts and *Planorbis* or *Bulinus* species water snails as IHs (147c – see page 243). Development of free-living stages and asexual multiplication in snails is similar to the life cycle of *Fasciola hepatica*. Metacercariae ingested with herbage excyst in the duodenum of the final host. Young flukes attach to and feed on plugs of duodenal mucosal tissue for about 6 weeks before migrating to the ventral forestomach, where they mature. The prepatent period is about 8 weeks and, under favourable conditions, development in the snail takes about 4 weeks.
**ii.** Adult flukes are often present in large numbers in the rumen and reticulum, but do not cause clinical disease. Heavy infection by immature flukes in the duodenum causes erosion of the duodenal mucosa and has been associated with diarrhoea, inappetence and dehydration in young calves. Disease may also occur while the parasite migrates from the duodenum to the rumen and reticulum along the submucosal lining of the omasum and abomasum. Co-infection with *Salmonella dublin* and *Salmonella typhimurium* has been reported, although the role of paramphistomes in triggering disease associated with salmonellosis is unclear.

**148 i.** How can a diagnosis of the parasite disease described in case **147** be confirmed in live animals?
**ii.** How can this parasitic infection be treated and controlled?

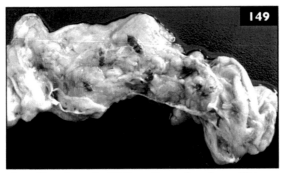

**149** In a sheep breeding farm in Heilongjiang Province, China, animals of one flock show anorexia, recumbency and depression. One of the affected animals dies and post-mortem examination reveals these abnormal structures in the pancreatic duct (**149**).
**i.** What abnormality can be seen?
**ii.** How do sheep become infected with this parasite?
**iii.** Would the clinical signs exhibited by the sheep be associated with infection by this parasite?
**iv.** What measures can be taken to prevent this infection?

**148 i.** Examination of a faecal sedimentation preparation for the presence of the characteristic paramphistome eggs can be used to confirm prepatent infection, but is of little value for diagnosis of disease caused by migrating larval stages. The egg is roughly oval, thin-shelled, about 150 µm long and operculate, similar to *F. hepatica* eggs. Unlike *F. hepatica* eggs, which are brown due to bile staining, *P. cervi* eggs are clear (**148**).

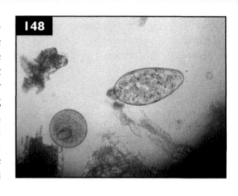

**ii.** Resorantel and oxyclozanide are reported to be effective for treatment of both immature and adult *P. cervi*, although neither is licensed for use in the UK. Evasive management strategies are not straightforward in countries where the epidemiology of paramphistomes is not fully understood, such as in the UK. The IH snails require a permanent water source, from which they are dispersed by flooding and heavy rainfall. Cercarial production by the snails occurs when the water levels recede, making the metacercariae available to grazing ruminants. The situation is complicated by aestivation of the snails when the water masses dry out and their reactivation following rainfall.

**149 i.** Digenetic flukes of the genus *Eurytrema* (e.g. *E. pancreaticum*), which live in pancreatic ducts of ruminants in parts of Asia, Brazil and Venezuela.
**ii.** There are two consecutive IHs, a land snail followed by a grasshopper. Infection of the definitive host (sheep) occurs via ingestion of a grasshopper infected by the larval stage. The flukes then migrate from the small intestine to the pancreatic duct.
**iii.** *Eurytrema* is not a serious threat unless the animal is severely infected. Mildly infected sheep do not generally show obvious clinical signs, but severely infected sheep exhibit poor condition, emaciation, indigestion, depression, anaemia, submandibular oedema, diarrhoea and mucus in faeces. The presence of *E. pancreaticum* in the pancreatic ducts causes inflammation and scar tissue formation in some areas of the pancreas.
**iv.** Control of infection is difficult due to the longevity of *E. pancreaticum* eggs and the wide distribution of the IHs. Preventive measures include routine deworming and reducing exposure to the IHs. *Eurytrema* species are zoonotic, therefore prevention of human infection is very significant.

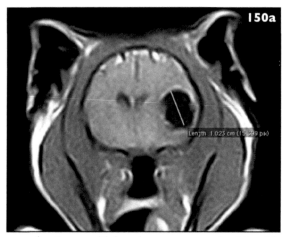

150 An MRI scan of a 7-year-old female cat presented with a history of circling and behavioural changes is shown (150a).

i. Describe the imaging abnormalities.

ii. What is the differential diagnosis?

iii. What other diagnostic tests should be carried out to establish a definitive diagnosis?

iv. How common is this problem in cats, and is it a problem in humans?

v. How should this patient be managed?

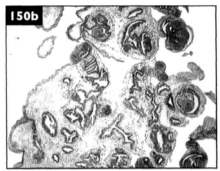

150 i. There is a spherical lesion approximately 1 cm in diameter of T1 hypointensity/T2 hyperintensity within the forebrain on the left side.

ii. Includes neoplasia (meningioma is the most common intracranial neoplasm in cats), a parasite cyst and infectious meningomyelitis. Based on the clinical history and MRI appearance, the cystic brain lesion is suggestive of 'gid or sturdy'.

iii. Histopathological examination of the resected cyst revealed scolices growing on the internal layer (150b), a feature highly suggestive of larvae of some taeniid species (e.g. *Coenurus serialis, C. cerebralis*). These species can use the cat as an IH, therefore differentiation among them is necessary. *Taenia serialis* and *T. multiceps* can be differentiated on a morphological basis, but to date little work has been done to differentiate them at the molecular level. The coenurus found in this case is likely to be *C. serialis* because of the linearly distributed scolices (characteristic of *C. serialis*, the larva of *T. serialis*).

iv. Reports of cerebral coenurosis in cats are uncommon. However, CNS infection with *Coenurus* has been reported in many human cases, especially children, who become IHs of *T. multiceps* after ingesting its eggs. The occurrence of coenurosis in this cat indicates that *T. multiceps* is capable of crossing the species barrier in this geographic locality and its larval development can occur in unusual hosts; this may constitute a zoonotic risk, especially for immunocompromised humans. For these reasons, feline cerebral coenurosis should be given more consideration even if the number of reported cases in cats is small.

v. By surgical removal of the cyst followed by prophylactic antibiotics and administration of mebendazole, albendazole or praziquantel. Corticosteroids can be given to reduce pericystic oedema within the brain.

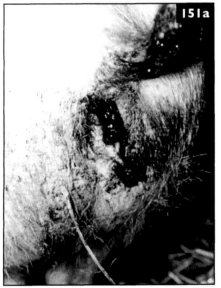

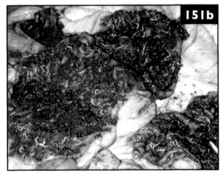

151 Groups of fattener pigs (50–120 kg) are being raised in both indoor and outdoor pens. Occasional pigs have voluminous soft faeces with specks of blood and mucus (151a). Close examination of the partially washed colon of one affected runt pig at necropsy shows nematode worms protruding from the mucosa (151b).
i. What is the name of this parasite? Describe its life cycle, and compare it with that of other porcine nematodes.
ii. Discuss treatment and control options for this parasite in outdoor pigs.

152 You are called to a poultry farm where the owner suspects he has a problem with coccidial infection.
i. What types of protozoa cause avian coccidiosis?
ii. Describe the signs of coccidial infection that you might observe in the flock.

151 i. *Trichuris suis*, the common whipworm. Variations in thickness of the anterior and posterior segments give the parasite its characteristic 'whip-like' appearance. Like *Ascaris suum*, the life cycle of *T. suis* is direct and does not require any IH in the environment. However, unlike *A. suum* larvae, *T. suis* larvae do not migrate extraintestinally and therefore there are no respiratory tract or liver lesions. Whipworm eggs (151c) are oval and yellow-brown with bipolar plugs. Eggs are passed in faeces from infected animals. They are single celled and not infectious for 1–2 months. Like *A. suum*, these eggs are highly resistant and can remain viable in outdoor conditions for several years. Ingested eggs are partially digested and larvae penetrate and develop in the large intestine mucosa. The adult worm's thicker posterior one-third then emerges through the mucosal surface into the lumen, while the thin anterior two-thirds remains embedded in the mucosal layers. The prepatent period is 6–8 weeks.

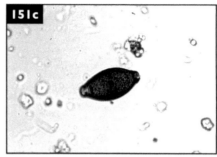

ii. Pasture rotation and properly timed anthelmintic treatment reduce contamination. Eggs stay in the upper 300 mm of soil. Clinical cases in pastured pigs require a large infectious dose, so cases tend to be sporadic unless pigs are kept for long periods in a small area. Groups of pigs may be treated for *A. suum* with piperazine, but this is not effective against *Trichuris*. Other anthelmintic products, including ivermectin, doramectin, flubendazole, fenbendazole, dichlorvos and levamisole, are generally effective against *Trichuris*.

152 i. At least nine species of *Eimeria* (phylum Apicomplexa, family Eimeriidae) occur in chickens and six are important (*E. acervulina*, *E. maxima*, *E. brunette*, *E. necatrix*, *E. mitis* and *E. tenella*). All chicken *Eimeria* species are host specific and tissue tropic (occur in particular parts of the intestine). For example, *E. tenella* infections are found only in the caeca.

ii. Birds will show loss of appetite, emaciation and weight loss, weakness and diarrhoea. Deep tissue invading species such as *E. maxima*, *E. necatrix* and *E. tenella* cause severe necrosis, haemorrhage of the intestinal mucosa and bloody diarrhoea and may result in death.

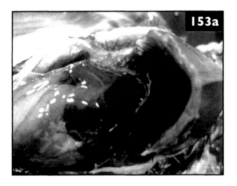

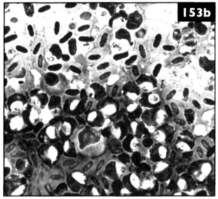

153 A breeder of canaries and native finches is experiencing heavy mortality among recently fledged birds. The birds are often found dead with no previous signs of illness; some have exhibited respiratory signs shortly prior to death. The breeder submits a recently deceased goldfinch for post-mortem examination. The coelomic cavity (153a) and an impression smear of the liver (153b) are shown.
i. What is your diagnosis?
ii. What other lesions might you expect to find at necropsy? How can you diagnose this disease in live birds?
iii. What treatment would you advise?
iv. How would you advise the breeder on prevention in future years?

154 You are called to a free-range poultry farm to investigate the cause of death of some young birds. While at the farm you notice that some birds are extending their necks and appear to be gasping for breath. What is the most likely diagnosis, and how can the diagnosis be confirmed?

**153 i.** Atoxoplasmosis caused by *Isospora serini*.

**ii.** An enlarged, sometimes mottled liver, splenomegaly and oedematous small intestine are often found at necropsy. Impression smears of spleen and lungs in addition to the liver often reveal parasites within the cytoplasm of monocytes. Coccidia may occasionally be found in the faeces, but it is difficult to differentiate oocysts of *Isospora serini* from oocysts of intestinal *Isospora* species.

**iii.** Treatment of severely affected birds is usually unrewarding. Oocyst shedding may be suppressed by sulphachlorpyrazine in the drinking water for 5 days a week or toltrazuril for 2 consecutive days per week for several months until after the moult.

**iv.** Preventive measures include minimizing stress in adult breeding birds. This will boost birds immune system and in turn reduce faecal oocyst shedding. Reducing stress can be achieved by reducing stocking densities, ensuring good nutrition and employing good hygiene protocols.

**154** Infection by *Syngamus trachea*, a nematode that parasitizes the trachea of a wide range of birds. The disease is usually seen in young birds and in birds reared in outdoor pens. The related *Cyathostoma bronchialis* causes a similar condition in geese. Diagnosis is based initially on the classical clinical signs of 'gasping' and detection of eggs on faecal flotation, and confirmed on necropsy by finding adult worms in the characteristic position (i.e. adult males and females are present in a permanent copulation position forming a Y-shape [**154**]) in the posterior part of the trachea. *Syngamus* eggs should be discriminated from those of *Capillaria* species. *Syngamus* and *Capillaria* eggs both have bipolar plugs. However, *Syngamus* eggs are larger and contain several well-defined cells (morula) when passed in faeces (see **15**).

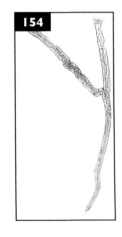

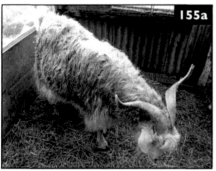
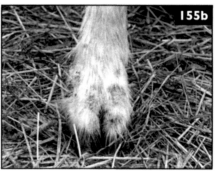

155 An adult male Cashmere goat is presented with severe exudative dermatitis affecting the entire body. The overlying hair is wet to touch, discoloured and matted (155a). The animal is extremely pruritic and in poor body condition. Several other animals in the herd are also pruritic. Many are seen nibbling their feet and the skin of their limbs distal to the accessory digits is covered by dry, crusty scabs (155b).
i. What is the most likely cause of this severe skin disease, and how can the diagnosis be confirmed?
ii. How can this problem be managed?

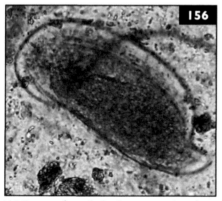

156 This organism (156) was found during a routine faecal screen of an adult Russian tortoise.
i. What is the organism?
ii. Is it significant?
iii. How would you treat this tortoise?

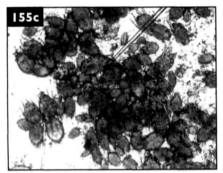
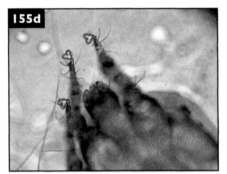

**155 i.** Chorioptic mange caused by *Chorioptes caprae*. *C. caprae* and *C. ovis* are specific host-adapted synonyms of *C. bovis*. The mites feed on epidermal debris, causing exudative dermatitis. The skin lesions are a mite-induced hypersensitivity reaction. Diagnosis is confirmed by microscopical examination of superficial skin scrapes or clear adhesive tape applied to the edges of distinct lesions. *C. bovis* are 0.25–0.50 mm long, oval-shaped mites (**155c**). They are identified as *Chorioptes* by their rounded mouthparts, short unjointed pedicels and bell-shaped suckers (**155d**). The anterior epimeres run more or less parallel. Mites tend to form clusters, so failure to find them in skin scrapes from individual animals with obvious lesions does not rule out a diagnosis of chorioptic mange.

**ii.** Treatment in goats is problematic because topical treatments may fail to penetrate to the skin because of matting of the overlying hair. There is little information available regarding the efficacy or safety of endectocide drugs used under the prescribing cascade.

**156 i.** *Nyctotherus* species, a ciliate protozoan.

**ii.** *Nyctotherus* is generally considered to be a normal commensal of the GI tract of tortoises and is frequently encountered in faeces. It may be pathogenic in high numbers.

**iii.** Generally, treatment is not necessary. High numbers of *Nyctotherus* are often associated with an inappropriately high level of fruit in the diet and numbers reduce when fruit is eliminated from the diet. Metronidazole is effective if treatment is needed.

**157** What are the consequences of infestation with *Chorioptes caprae* in a sheep flock (see also case **155**).

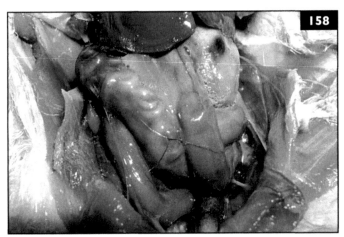

**158** Several birds of prey from a private collection housed outdoors have progressive weight loss, anorexia and diarrhoea. The birds are fed fresh pigeons. Repeated antiprotozoal treatments administered by the owner are not effective and after 1 month, one Eurasian sparrowhawk dies. Gross necropsy reveals complete occlusion of the intestine by roundworms immediately visible through the intestinal wall (**158**). Faecal flotation testing is negative for coccidia and other protozoan parasites.
i. What is your diagnosis?
ii. How common is this infection in cage and aviary birds?
iii. How would you manage the remainder of the collection?

157 *C. bovis* infestation causes low-grade pruritus and exudative dermatitis over the poll, above the coronary bands, around the accessory digits (157a) and over the pasterns of the hindlimbs of ewes and rams, and on the scrotum of rams. Lesions on the limbs and poll are of little clinical significance, but severe mange affecting more than one-third of the scrotum can raise the temperature of the testes and is an important cause of impaired spermatogenesis and poor reproductive performance. Scrotal mange is characterized by superficial, exudative, fissured and haemorrhagic lesions, with some serous exudation and matting and staining of any overlying wool on the lower third of the scrotum (157b). Handling of the scrotum often initiates a nibble response. Thickening and fissuring of the scrotal skin, without evidence of scab formation or bleeding, is a common finding, particularly when rams have previously been winter housed, and is not necessarily indicative of scrotal mange. In some cases these lesions might be associated with skin penetration by infective *Strongyloides papillosus* larvae.

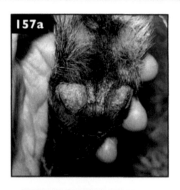

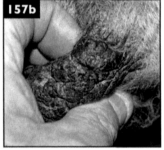

158 i. The most likely diagnosis, based on the high intensity of infection, location of the worms in the small intestine and the roundworm morphology, is ascarid infection.

ii. Ascaridiosis is one of the most common roundworm infections in birds housed in outdoor aviaries. Access to the ground is the most important source of ascarid egg ingestion.

iii. By performing a parasitological screening on a regular basis (at least 2–3 times every year). Ascarid eggs are resistant to common disinfectants, therefore cleaning the ground by physical removal of the dirty surface layer by means of steam is recommended.

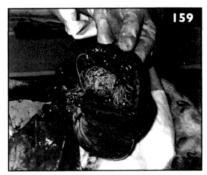

**159** A 7-year-old Boxer dog is referred to your clinic and a diagnosis of heartworm disease is made. The owner elects euthanasia and permits a necropsy. Diagnosis is confirmed on post-mortem examination (**159**).
i. What are 'heartworms'?
ii. Describe the typical clinical signs in dogs.
iii. How is this disease diagnosed in the live animal?
iv. How can this disease be prevented?

**160** Flea infestations are common and elimination can be expensive and time-consuming.
i. How can you determine whether fleas on a pet are coming from the outdoor environment or from inside the home?
ii. When would you spray your home with an IGR, and what does this do?

**159 i.** Filarial parasites (*Dirofilaria immitis*) that are spread from host to host through the bites of mosquitoes. The definitive host is the dog, but cats, wolves, coyotes, foxes, other animals and humans can also be infected.

**ii.** Adult worms reside in the pulmonary arterial system and cause damage to the lung vessels and tissue. Occasionally, adult heartworms migrate to the right side of the heart and even the great veins entering the heart in heavy infections. Infected dogs may show exercise intolerance, decreased appetite, loss of weight, cough and listlessness. Animals with severe heartworm disease will show lack of endurance during exercise and in rare situations they may die of sudden heart failure.

**iii.** By one or more of the following approaches: morphological identification of circulating microfilariae (mf) via direct blood smear, modified Knott's test or after millipore filtration of blood; histochemical or immunohistochemical staining of circulating mf; serological testing (a patient-side heartworm test kit with 99.2% sensitivity and 100% specificity is commercially available); through molecular approaches; radiography to evaluate the severity of lung damage caused by the presence of worms.

**iv.** Chemoprophylaxis is nearly 100% effective in preventing heartworm infection when administered appropriately. Several drugs are available. MLs (ivermectin, milbemycin oxime, moxidectin, selamectin) are the drugs of choice for chemoprophylaxis in dogs. All the chemoprophylaxis medications are microfilaricidal when administered continuously over a period of time. Some MLs may also have an adulticidal effect if used continuously for a prolonged period.

**160 i.** If the owner has bites around the ankles, this is a sure sign that the infestation is coming from inside the home. Some people are less sensitive to bites than others, so if the owners have not noticed bites, this does not rule out an internal infestation. If the pet has more than 10 fleas on it, it is more likely that the pupae are indoors than outdoors.

**ii.** With a household infestation, the pet should be treated with a veterinary flea product. Meanwhile application of an IGR will prevent existing eggs in the environment from developing into larvae and prevent larvae developing into pupae. No insecticide kills the pupae because they are buried deep in the pile of the carpet, in cracks and crevices in the floor or within soft furnishings and are protected by their cocoon, which in turn is covered in debris. Once the pupae hatch, the newly emerged fleas will jump onto the treated pet and die.

161 A 9-week-old female Norfolk Terrier is presented with pruritus and excessive dorsal scaling (161). The puppy was purchased from a breeder 2 weeks previously. The owner reports pruritic papular lesions on both of her forearms. The puppy's limbs and ventrum are unaffected, although a bilateral ceruminous otitis externa is noted.

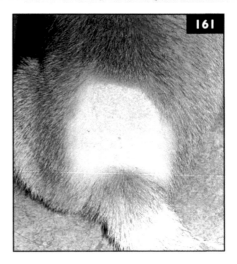

i. What is your differential diagnosis?
ii. What diagnostic tests would you perform?
iii. Is this condition specific to dogs?
iv. What are the appropriate treatment options?

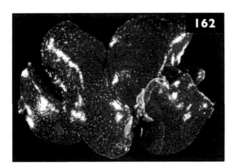

162 A rabbit breeder has had increased mortality among her young stock over the past 3 months, which happen to coincide with the summer months and hot weather. She estimates that approximately 25% of rabbits 3–6 months of age have decreased appetites and poor weight gain, and about 20% of these animals eventually die. The rabbits are raised in wooden hutches with wire floors, in a small building behind the breeder's home. One 9-week-old female rabbit, which died recently, is submitted to a diagnostic laboratory for necropsy. Findings include emaciation and small nodular lesions in the liver (162).

i. What is the likely diagnosis, and what agent causes this disease?
ii. What would you expect to see histologically in tissue sections containing the liver lesions?

**161 i.** Pruritic papular lesions on the owner are compatible with a diagnosis of cheyletiellosis, although flea infestation, otodectic mange and scabies should also be considered. Less likely differentials include pediculosis, primary seborrhoea, malnutrition and demodicosis.

**ii.** Examination of debris from a coat brushing, preferably onto a dark surface, using a hand lens. Low-power microscopical examination of superficial skin scrapings in liquid paraffin or acetate tape preparations from the skin surface may allow identification of the mite. Large numbers of eggs, nymphal stages and adult mites of *Cheyletiella yasguri* can be detected by these techniques. Similarly, examination of ear wax using a hand lens or microscope may reveal *Otodectes cynotis* mites, as in this case.

**iii.** No, cheyletiellosis is found in dogs, cats and rabbits. *Cheyletiella yasguri* is the species found on dogs, although there is no host specificity. All species can transiently affect in-contact humans. Puppies and kittens, particularly those from breeding establishments, appear most susceptible.

**iv.** Insecticidal efficacy does not always equate to acaricidal efficacy, and baths may be more effective than low-volume aerosols in reaching mites that are protected by surface scale. Selenium sulphide 1% is frequently used for the treatment of cheyletiellosis. Amitraz, phosmet and ivermectin have also been used. Use of a 0.25% fipronil spray has recently been reported. Affected and in-contact animals should be treated for 6–8 weeks and regular use of an effective environmental flea control product is recommended.

**162 i.** Based on the clinical history and necropsy findings, this rabbit had hepatic coccidiosis caused by *Eimeria stiedae*.

**ii.** The nodular white to pale yellow foci are areas of biliary epithelial hyperplasia and hypertrophy. In addition, there is usually some degree of chronic inflammation (cholangitis: inflammation of bile ductules), with infiltration of lymphocytes, macrophages and plasma cells, in affected portal triads.

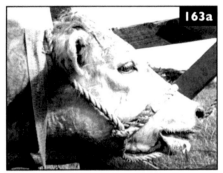

**163** A 7-year-old cow is presented with coughing, dyspnoea, respiratory distress (**163a**), weight loss, reduced milk yield and unthriftiness. A diagnosis of lungworm (*D. viviparus*) disease is made based on the history, character and nature of the dyspnoea and the failure of antibiotic therapy to ameliorate the condition. How can a definitive diagnosis of lungworm disease be achieved?

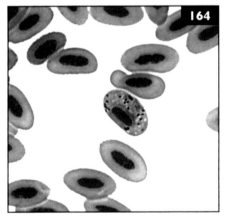

**164** During assessment of a grounded wild hobby, you examine a blood smear and find several erythrocytes containing intracytoplasmic inclusions that appear to wrap around the erythrocyte nucleus without displacing it (**164**).

**i.** What are these inclusions?
**ii.** Are they significant?
**iii.** What clinical signs might you expect to see?
**iv.** If you decide to treat this condition, what would you use?

163 Presumptive diagnosis is based on clinical signs, grazing history and knowledge of the patterns of parasite epidemiology. However, clinical signs of this disease are not pathognomonic and are often confused with bacterial or viral pneumonia. Therefore, lungworm disease should be included in the differential diagnosis for persistent respiratory manifestations in cows, especially in enzootic areas. Definitive diagnosis can be made after the demonstration of L1s in faeces using the Baermann technique. However, L1s may be absent if this was reinfection syndrome. Tracheal washes may provide cytological evidence of eosinophilic inflammation consistent

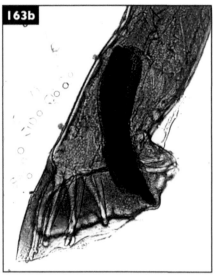

with parasitic bronchitis or pneumonia. Bronchoscopy and radiography may be helpful. Serological tests have been developed based on crude or somatic antigens of *D. viviparus*. However, serology may fail to differentiate between recent and past infection, or to detect antibodies during the prepatent period. Also, seroprevalence rates do not always accurately reflect the presence of clinical disease. Confirmation of diagnosis is made by the detection of adult nematodes in the bronchi and trachea at post-mortem examination. Adult lungworms are long, thin white worms with small buccal cavities. Males are 17–50 mm in length; females 23–80 mm. A small copulatory bursa with characteristic spicules can be seen in males (163b).

164 i. *Haemoproteus* species gametocytes, which contain refractile iron pigments and often encircle more than half of the erythrocyte's nucleus without displacing it.
ii. *Haemoproteus* is common in wild raptors and is generally of low pathogenicity.
iii. Ill-thrift, exercise intolerance, anorexia and haemolytic anaemia, especially if the bird is immunocompromised. Harris' Hawks, Tawny Owls and Snowy Owls may be more susceptible to severe disease.
iv. Chloroquine, mefloquine and primaquine have been reported to reduce parasitaemia in some cases.

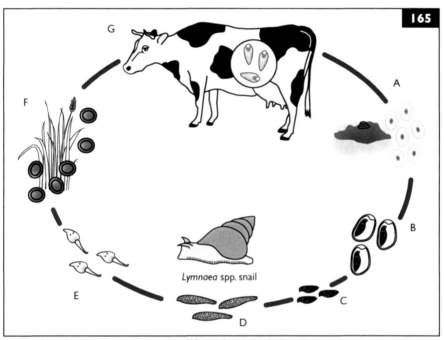

165 i. To which parasite does this life cycle (165) belong?
ii. Name and describe each of the lettered stages.
iii. What is the clinical significance of this parasite?
iv. What are the treatment options for this parasite?

**165 i.** Liver flukes of the genus *Fasciola*.

**ii.** (A) Immature eggs shed in manure; (B) eggs mature and embryos hatch; (C) miracidia; (D) rediae; (E) cercariae; (F) cercariae encyst on grass into metacercariae (infective stage); (G) adult flukes reach sexual maturity in liver and gallbladder of the definitive host.

**iii.** *Fasciola* species are of considerable importance in the veterinary and agri-food sectors, especially in temperate regions of the world. Fasciolosis is a significant zoonotic infection of humans, with upward of 180 million people at risk of infection. Climatic changes may favour transmission of the developmental stages of the parasite within the IH (snails), so prevalence is anticipated to increase further.

**iv.** Triclabendazole (TCBZ) is the mainstay of chemotherapy against liver fluke infection. It is a benzimidazole with fasciolicidal activity against *Fasciola hepatica*, *F. gigantica*, *F. magna* and *Paragonimus* species, but not against cestodes or nematodes. It is the only drug that can target the migratory juvenile stages from just 2 days post infection through to the mature adult flukes, thus offering effective control for both acute and chronic fasciolosis. However, overuse has led to the development of drug resistance in some fluke populations. Synergistic combinations of drugs with two mechanisms of actions (e.g. TCBZ plus clorsulon and TCBZ plus luxabendazole) have been used in an effort to slow the development of resistance.

**166** Individuals within a group of 30-kg pigs on a small family farm show continual rubbing of the body against the sides of pens, frequent head shaking and the occurrence of aural haematomas. Closer examination shows waxy, dark brown encrustations within the ears, encrusted elbows and scurfy, dirty hindlimbs. Numerous ear and skin scrapings are collected and occasional microscopic parasites are noted in one or two samples (**166a**).

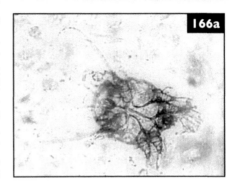

i. What is this parasite?
ii. Is this diagnosis easy to make via skin scrapings?
iii. What secondary effects or sequelae can occur in infected pigs?

**167** A 2-year-old male lovebird is presented with feather picking, weight loss, diarrhoea and skin irritation (**167**). Faecal flotation using a commercial sodium nitrate solution does not reveal any parasite eggs. However, a second flotation with a zinc sulphate solution prepared to a specific gravity of 1.18 allows the detection of several oval to ellipsoid, 10 µm organisms. A direct smear of a faecal dropping at 100x magnification reveals tiny, fast moving, pear-shaped 15 µm organisms.

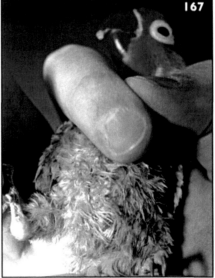

i. What is described in the faecal flotation and direct faecal smear? Does this explain the clinical signs seen in the lovebird?
ii. Why is zinc sulphate solution superior in the identification of this organism?
iii. Why are mobile microorganisms seen only in fresh direct faecal smears?
iv. Is this infection zoonotic?

**166 i.** Pig mange mite, *Sarcoptes scabei* var *suis*. Mites burrow into the skin and lay eggs in tunnels in the skin, which causes severe host irritation and pruritus.
**ii.** Reliable and sensitive diagnosis is the main problem for adequate control and eradication programmes. Definitive diagnosis of swine scabies is not always easy because of the minute size of the parasite and its intracutaneous localization.
**iii.** This mite continues to cause problems for the pig industry worldwide despite the availability of effective treatments (e.g. ivermectin). Aural haematomas can occur

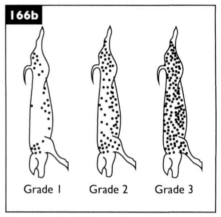

due to the pig frequently shaking its head and ears, and middle ear damage can result. Other sequelae include greasy pig disease (*Staphylococcus hyicus*), which flourishes in damaged skin, and papular dermatitis, which is part of an allergic host skin response commonly seen in pigs with mange. Large numbers of small red papules occur over the body and persist for long periods. This reaction forms the basis of a slaughter facility check for mange (i.e. grading the severity of papular dermatitis at slaughter using a 0 to 3 scale for classifying carcasses, **166b**).

**167 i.** Based on the morphometric characteristics of the organisms detected, this bird is probably infected with *Giardia* species, a flagellate protozoan. *Giardia* infection is mainly associated with diarrhoea in several species of animal, and in the Class Aves giardiosis is also frequently related to feather picking and skin irritation. It is quite common in several species of psittacines such as lovebirds, cockatiels and budgerigars.
**ii.** Sodium nitrate solution distorts *Giardia* cysts very rapidly, whereas zinc sulphate solution maintains the parasite morphology and, therefore, facilitates its identification.
**iii.** *Giardia* trophozoites do not survive for a long time away from the host and their motility is also affected by temperature.
**iv.** The role of avian hosts in the transmission of *Giardia* to humans is not well documented.

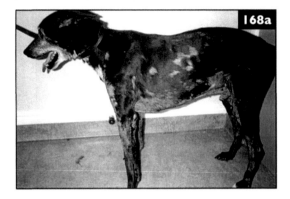

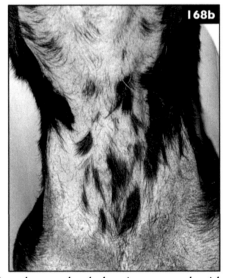

168 A 14-year-old male crossbred dog is presented with generalized patchy alopecia affecting particularly the ventral neck, chest, abdomen and limbs (168a, b). Pruritus is reported to be mild. Erythema and crusting are present on the medial thighs. Tufts of hair are easily epilated from affected areas. Mild scaling and comedones are also noted in these areas.

i. What is your suspected diagnosis, and how would you confirm this?
ii. What is your differential diagnosis in this case?
iii. How would you treat this dog?

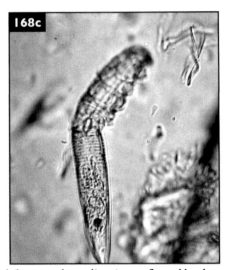

**168 i.** Generalized, adult-onset demodicosis, confirmed by demonstrating *Demodex* mites (**168c**) in deep skin scrapings or hair pluckings from affected areas, examined initially under low power. (**Note:** *Demodex* mites can be present in small numbers in normal dogs, but detection of even one mite should alert the clinician to search for more by further sampling.)

**ii.** Dermatophytosis, pyoderma, drug eruption, dermatomyositis.

**iii.** This is a challenging canine skin disease to treat. Reported cure rates for topical amitraz vary from 0–92% and may be influenced by the concentration and frequency of application of the solution. Treatment may be aided by bathing the dog in a 2.5% benzoyl peroxide shampoo, towel drying and then applying a 0.05% amitraz solution. This is repeated weekly for 12 weeks. A systemic antibacterial drug (e.g. cephalexin) may be administered orally for the first 3–6 weeks to resolve concurrent pyoderma. Weekly amitraz bathing should be continued for 3 weeks beyond negative skin scrapings. Avermectins are of value in the management of demodicosis, used either solely or in addition to amitraz. Ivermectin is contradicted in Collies and related cross-breeds as it can cause potentially fatal idiosyncratic reactions.

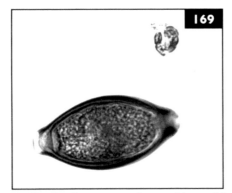

169 A captive baboon collection has an ongoing problem with diarrhoea, lethargy, abdominal pain, weight loss, inappetence and dehydration. An egg is observed on faecal flotation (169).
i. What is this egg?
ii. What anthelmintic should be recommended for treatment?

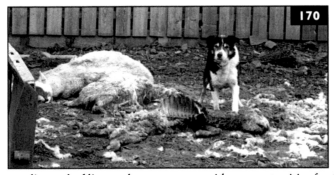

170 Improper disposal of livestock carcasses provides opportunities for farm dogs to gain access to carcasses and become infested with various parasites (170). It is commonplace for farm dogs to be kept in parts of buildings that are subsequently used for sheep housing. What are the potential sheep parasitic disease threats posed by these practices?

**169 i.** The distinctive oval shape with a thick brown shell and plugs at both ends are specific features of eggs of the nematode *Trichuris trichiura*. This species infects the large intestine and caecum of captive and wild primates as well as humans. Different *Trichuris* species affect various domestic animal species (e.g. *T. vulpis* in dogs, *T. suis* in swine).
**ii.** Fenbendazole (50 mg/kg PO for 3 consecutive days) can be very effective.

**170 (1)** Sarcocystosis. Dogs are the definitive hosts for *Sarcocystis tenella* and *S. arieticanis*, and sheep are IHs. Sheep ingest sporocysts from feed or pasture contaminated by dog faeces. Sarcocysts (cystic stage) are found in heart and skeletal muscles of most sheep, but outbreaks of clinical disease only occur when the environmental challenge is high. Sarcocysts within the brain and spinal cord are a common cause of vague neurological disease including generalized tremors, compulsive nibbling and recumbency, and fore- or hindlimb paralysis in 6–12-month-old lambs.

**(2)** Neosporosis. *Neospora caninum* is a closely related protozoal parasite to *Toxoplasma gondii* and is an important cause of abortion in dairy cattle. The definitive host for *N. caninum* is the dog, which sheds oocysts. Recognized IHs are cattle and horses. Abortions and birth of congenitally infected lambs have been demonstrated following experimental infection during the early stages of pregnancy, but it is not known if comparable levels of challenge can occur under field conditions.

**(3)** Tapeworms. Dogs and/or wild canids are definitive hosts for the cestode parasites *Taenia hydatigena* (*Cysticercus tenuicollis*), *Taenia multiceps* (coenurosis), *Taenia ovis* (*Cysticercus ovis*) and *Echinococcus granulosus* (hydatidosis), which can cause clinical disease, result in downgrading or condemnation of carcasses or present serious human health risks. Sheep and other IHs are usually infected when they ingest tapeworm eggs containing oncospheres from pasture contaminated by infected canid faeces. Oncospheres then penetrate the gut wall of the IH and travel via the blood to different target organs, where they develop into metacestodes (cysticercus, coenurus, hydatid), which occupy normal tissue and may result in clinical disease.

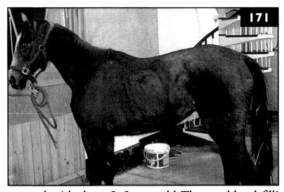

**171** You are presented with three 2–3-year-old Thoroughbred fillies that are kept in a closed yard with 47 other horses. The three horses are losing weight and are weak. They have been dewormed every 8 weeks with ivermectin and were treated with 'double-dose' pyrantel in the autumn. Worm egg counts taken 6 weeks prior to your examination of the animals were negative. The horses were reported to have had intermittent, self-limiting diarrhoea over the past 6–8 weeks and have been lying down for a considerable amount of time each day. Over the past week, one of the horses became so weak that it could barely stand (**171**). The horse was euthanized and post-mortem examination recovered approximately 200 litres of adult *Parascaris equorum* parasites.

**i.** Why did these horses become weak and thin?
**ii.** What other clinical signs can be associated with infection with these parasites?
**iii.** How could these horses have such massive infections of *P. equorum* with no worm egg counts on faecal flotation?
**iv.** Why did these horses have such massive infections when they were being dewormed so aggressively?

**171 i.** The likely reason is that the worm burden was such that the energy being consumed was not being absorbed due to the physical intestinal obstruction caused by these parasites. In addition, the parasites consume the liquid contents in the intestine, further robbing the horse of nutrients.

**ii.** Clinical signs are usually associated with the migration of L4s, which migrate through the lungs causing coughing in young horses (usually <1 year). In severe cases the pulmonary phase can be associated with secondary bacterial infection and, occasionally, bleeding into the airways. In addition, this condition can be associated with clinical signs of abdominal pain caused by physical obstruction of the small intestine by the parasites, which can rarely lead to intestinal rupture.

**iii.** The prepatent period of *P. equorum* is approximately 3–4 months, therefore it is possible that when these horses were sampled they had large worm burdens, but the worms were not yet producing ova (prepatent infection). Also, if faeces are examined when horses have diarrhoea, there can be a dilutional effect on those ova that are present, so the worm burden and number of ova actually being produced can be underestimated.

**iv.** Either the worm burden was so high that they were largely protected from the action of the drugs administered, or the parasites were resistant to the anthelmintics administered.

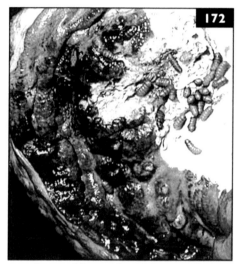

172 The gastric mucosa from a 10-month-old Quarter horse colt is shown (172).
i. What parasites are pictured here?
ii. What are the major clinical effects of these parasites?
iii. What are the main pathological effects or lesions caused by these parasites?
iv. What type(s) of anthelmintics would be effective against these parasites?

173 How can the protozoal and cestode disease threats discussed in case 170 be averted?

**172 i.** Larvae of botflies (*Gasterophilus* species). Three species of botfly are distributed worldwide: *G. intestinalis* (common bot), *G. haemorrhoidalis* (nose or lip bot) and *G. nasalis* (throat bot).

**ii.** Even with large numbers, there are usually no clinical signs associated with bots. Owners may notice the small, cream coloured eggs on the hairs of the legs or throat.

**iii.** The oral hooks of the larvae may cause erosions or ulcerations in the GI mucosa, and these lesions may heal with raised rims of hyperplastic mucosal epithelium or fibrosis. Oral stages of the larvae may cause tracts lined by purulent exudate in the gingiva.

**iv.** Avermectins are effective against oral and gastric stages of the bots. Moxidectin is effective against gastric stages. Current recommendations are for at least two treatments annually, one in the early spring, when the first bot eggs are seen on the hair coat, and one toward the end of the fly season. In locations where the botfly season may be long, additional treatments may be necessary.

**173** By preventing dogs and wild canids from having access to sheep carcasses. They should be kept in a secure area while awaiting removal. Feed stores should be kept biosecure (**173**), in particular ensuring that it is impossible for dogs to enter and defecate in them. Dogs that may have access to areas in which sheep are kept should be treated with a cestocide every 6–8 weeks. Praziquantel is effective against all the common dog tapeworms, including *E. granulosus*, while nitroscanate is effective against *T. ovis* and *T. hydatigena*, but not against *E. granulosus*. Dogs should be confined for 48 hours after treatment and any infected faeces collected and carefully disposed of. Meat or offal fed to farm dogs should either be thoroughly cooked to 56°C (133°F) or frozen to –10°C (14°F) for 10 days to ensure death of the larval cysts. On many farms, attempts to disrupt the sheep-to-dog life cycle of cestodes and *Sarcocystis* species are hindered by public access and dog walking activity.

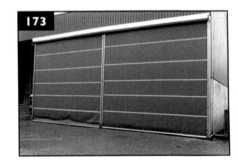

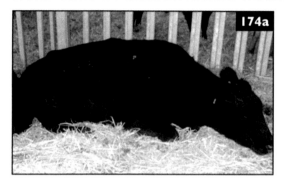

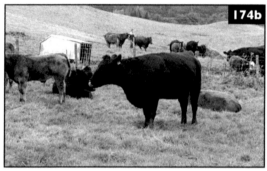

174 In early September (northern hemisphere), coughing is noted in 6-month-old spring-born calves in a herd of 250 beef suckler cows. The cattle are grazed in groups of 20 and 40 with their calves in different enclosed fields on an upland farm. During mid-September, a 2.5-year-old Charolais-cross cow at pasture is seen with severe, acute respiratory disease; this cow dies the following morning. Two weeks later, another 2.5-year-old Charolais-cross cow, two 2.5-year-old Limousin-cross cows and a 3.5-year-old Limousin bull from the same group are presented with severe, acute-onset respiratory distress (174a). These animals display open-mouth breathing and moist coughs. It is mostly young cows in the group that are affected (174b), while older animals are unaffected. The affected group of cattle was grazed during August and the first 3 weeks of September on a field that had been ploughed and resown with grass two summers prior and thereafter was only periodically grazed by sheep. The cattle had been moved onto an adjacent field of mature grass just a few days before the main onset of respiratory disease.

i. List a differential diagnosis for this respiratory disease outbreak.
ii. How would you support a diagnosis of parasitic disease?
iii. How should the severely affected cattle be treated?

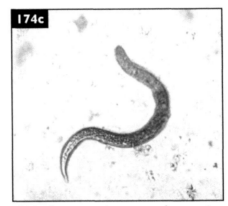

**174 i.** Parasitic bronchitis (lungworm), commonly seen in grazing cattle during the autumn. Fog fever: acute-onset pulmonary oedema rarely seen in the autumn after adult cows have been moved onto fast growing foggage or silage aftermath pastures. Bacterial infection (*Mycoplasma bovis*, *Mannheimia haemolytica* [less likely] or *Histophilus somni*). Viral infection (BVD, IBR, PI-3, BRSV).

**ii.** Identification of adventitious lung sounds on auscultation, particularly affecting the caudal lung fields, supported by finding L1 *Dictyocaulus viviparus* in Baermannized faecal samples (**174c**). Post-mortem examination of the cow that died revealed the presence of large numbers of *D. viviparus* in the bronchi and trachea and of parasitic pneumonia affecting adjacent parts of the lungs.

**iii.** Broad-spectrum anthelmintic administration is necessary, but could exacerbate the signs due to an allergic pneumonia if dead lungworms remain *in situ*. Therefore, levamisole, which paralyses lungworms rather than killing the larvae outright, is recommended. Corticosteroid therapy (not beyond the third month of pregnancy) is indicated, along with broad-spectrum antibiotic treatment of secondary bacterial infection.

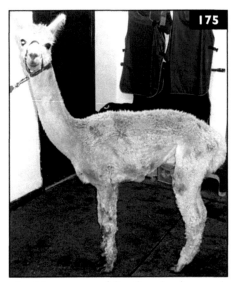

175 You are presented with a group of five female alpacas that are part of a herd of 30 animals that have shown signs of weight loss of 3 weeks' duration (175). Haematology reveals a moderate anaemia and a blood smear reveals inclusion bodies consistent with *Mycoplasma haemollamae*. Blood biochemistry profile reveals a significant increase in serum activities of GGT and ALP. Faecal worm egg count is negative except when faecal sedimentation is performed, and then a moderate number of fluke eggs are identified. A presumptive diagnosis of chronic disease caused by *Fasciola hepatica* is made.

i. Why is this animal anaemic?

ii. How does the diagnosis of *F. hepatica* differ in camelids compared with cattle?

iii. How can disease be treated and prevented?

**175 i.** Probably multifactorial in this case. *Fasciola hepatica* worms ingest and destroy red cells and there is likely to be a reduction in red cell production due to the underlying chronic disease process. In addition, South American camelids are often carriers of *M. haemollamae*, an intracellular organism affecting red cells. When animals become debilitated for other reasons, the number of *M. haemollamae* increases, which can also lead to red cell destruction.

**ii.** Diagnosis in cattle is based on history, physical examination (weight loss, anaemia, diarrhoea, submandibular oedema), increased liver damage indicators and decreased total protein and albumin concentrations. Faecal sedimentation can identify fluke eggs. There is also an ELISA that measures exposure to the parasite through measurement of antibodies in both serum and milk. All of these diagnostic methods can be used in alpacas, except for the ELISA, which is specific to cattle.

**iii.** As in ruminants, this disease requires ingestion of infective metacercariae that have developed within the mollusc *Lymnaea truncatula*. Preventing access to wet areas where these snails can propagate the disease is important in control. Treatment of affected individuals, and in-contact animals at risk of developing disease, involves administration of a flukicide (e.g. triclabendazole, albendazole, clorsulon).

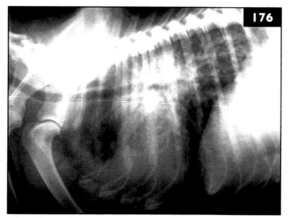

**176** A 6-year-old male Dalmatian is presented with a 1-month-history of cough and respiratory distress that does not respond to antibiotic therapy. A lateral thoracic radiograph is obtained (**176**).

**i.** Describe the radiographic abnormalities present.

**ii.** What is your differential diagnosis for these findings?

**iii.** What other tests are needed to distinguish between these diagnoses?

**iv.** Assuming the diagnosis is parasitic pneumonia, how can the disease be treated?

**v.** Is this parasitic disease zoonotic?

**176 i.** Multifocal bronchial and peribronchial interstitial and alveolar patterns associated with moderately dilated pulmonary arteries.

**ii.** Heartworm disease, *Angiostrongylus vasorum* infection, right-sided heart failure and right atrial haemangiosarcoma. Clinical signs and radiological findings indicate *A. vasorum* as the most likely cause. Radiographic changes seen in heartworm disease (right-sided cardiomegaly, enlarged main pulmonary artery, dilated and tortuous lobar pulmonary arteries, blunting of pulmonary arteries, enlarged caudal vena cava) are not present here. Also, heartworms that are obvious in the RV and RA as a mass of short parallel lines on echocardiography are not seen. There is no dilation of the RV. The cardiac silhouette was not abnormal (so a mass was not apparent).

**iii.** Detection and identification of L1s in faecal samples using the Baermann technique; cytological examination of tracheal wash or bronchoalveolar lavage; CBC; serological assays to rule out heartworm.

**iv.** With a variety of anthelmintic treatments (e.g. levamisole, ivermectin, fenbendazole). The treatment dose and length vary greatly and various protocols have shown differing degrees of success, due to the variable nature of the clinical signs. Supportive treatment with antibiotics, bronchodilators and corticosteroids is commonly given.

**v.** No cases of *A. vasorum* infection have been reported in humans; however, they can be infected with other *Angiostrongylus* species (e.g. *A. cantonensis*).

177 You examine a fresh wet-mount of a crop wash from a cockatiel displaying signs of lethargy, weight loss and regurgitation. Many motile organisms, with single long flagella, are visible. A dried, stained smear from the same cockatiel is shown (177). The cockatiel is one of a group housed in a small outdoor aviary.

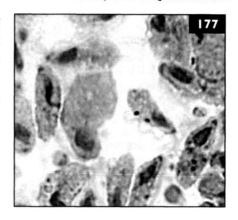

i. What are the organisms observed?
ii. How would you treat this individual?
iii. What preventive measures would you advise?

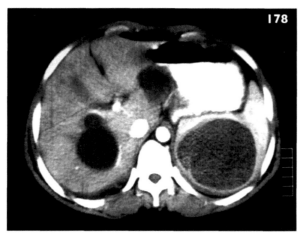

178 A 58-year-old man from a sheep-rearing area is seen by his physician because of an enlarged liver, with a palpable mass in the right upper quadrant of the abdomen. CT reveals a round space-occupying lesion in his liver (178).
i. Assuming the liver mass is parasite induced and based on the symptoms, what parasitic infection do you think this patient has probably contracted?
ii. How do humans become infected with this parasite?
iii. What risk to the patient exists during surgical removal of the cyst?
iv. How should this patient be treated?

**177 i.** *Trichomonas gallinae*, a motile protozoan parasite.
**ii.** With metronidazole, ronidazole or carnidazole.
**iii.** *T. gallinae* has a direct life cycle, being spread via contaminated food and water bowls and perches. Preventive measures include reducing stocking densities, ensuring food and water bowls are not placed under perches and regular cleaning and disinfection of perches and food bowls.

**178 i.** Hydatidosis, caused by *Echinococcus granulosus*. Microscopical examination of aspirated cyst fluid can reveal the presence of hydatid sand, a granular material consisting of free scolices and amorphous germinal material (see **69b**).
**ii.** *E. granulosus* eggs and proglottids are passed in dog faeces and ingested by humans. Eggs hatch, penetrate the intestinal wall, enter the circulation and form hydatid cysts in organs, especially the liver and lungs.
**iii.** During surgical removal and aspiration, fluid or tissue may leak out into the peritoneal cavity. Hydatid sand or bits of tissue may produce new cysts and cause disseminated infection. Spillage of hydatid fluid during open surgery has been shown to result in serious anaphylactic reaction.
**iv.** Surgical removal of the cystic lesion has a high success rate. Chemotherapy with benzimidazole compounds (mebendazole, albendazole) has also been used with some success to sterilize the cyst, decrease the chance of anaphylaxis and reduce the complications and recurrence rate postoperatively. In recent years, PAIR (puncture, aspiration, injection, re-aspiration) has been introduced and this is indicated for patients who cannot undergo surgery.

179 You are called in the spring to examine a flock of sheep in which four 6-week-old grazing lambs died unexpectedly. Post-mortem examination of the dead lambs reveals enteritis associated with very large numbers of adult nematodes in the small intestine. Some surviving lambs have scours, and faecal flotation reveals the presence of parasite eggs (**179**), despite the fact that the entire flock was recently treated with an anthelmintic.

i. What is your diagnosis?
ii. Why might you suspect *N. battus* rather than other GI nematodes?

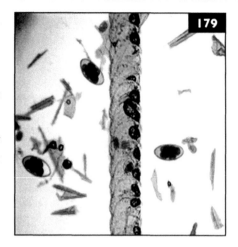

180 A 6-year-old neutered male DSH cat is presented with acute diarrhoea, vomiting, anorexia, lethargy, dyspnoea, dehydration and weakness. The cat is euthanized at the owner's request. This worm is found incidentally in the intestine (**180a**) and some eggs are detected in the faeces (**180b**).

i. What is your diagnosis?
ii. How do cats become infected with this parasite?
iii. How should this infection be treated and controlled?

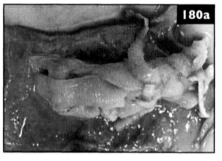

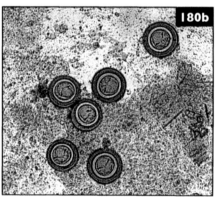

179 i. Based on the clinical history, faecal examination (characteristic egg size and morphology) and post-mortem examination of the lambs, the infection is due to *Nematodirus battus*.

ii. *N. battus* infection affects young lambs, causing considerable disease, especially among newly weaned lambs. Adult sheep are seldom or never affected. In addition, *Nematodirus* infection occurs in a restricted season (with specific environmental conditions) during which the majority of deaths occur. After a cold spring, any warmth in early summer encourages a mass hatch of eggs laid on pasture the previous year. *N. battus* hatches in response to an increase in environmental temperature following a period of chilling, resulting in a rapid increase in parasite infective stages on pasture over a short period of time. Hatching of larvae on pasture associated with rising temperatures increases the risk of disease in young lambs due to infection with *N. battus*. However, new reports suggest that some eggs hatch without a cold period. A change in the pattern of the disease has been reported with an increased autumn hatch of *Nematodirus*, which may reduce the numbers of eggs left to cause disease in spring, leading to an increase in autumn disease in lambs.

180 i. Tapeworm infection. Note the typical taeniid-type eggs (i.e. surrounded by a brown striated eggshell and containing a six-hooked embryo/embryophore). Based on the body segmentation of the worm, the characteristic features of the eggs and the location in the cat's intestine, this worm is most likely *Taenia taeniaformis*. Cats are the definitive host. Infected cats are asymptomatic, but motile proglottids may be seen in the faeces or on the perineal fur.

ii. From scavenging rodents (IH) in which the larval stage (*Cysticercus fasciolaris*) is present.

iii. Praziquantel is the most useful drug for cestodes and is effective at killing adult tapeworms. Some species require a higher dose (30–35 mg/kg) than the standard one (5–10 mg/kg). Drugs currently used to treat heartworm and other ectoparasite and endoparasite diseases are not effective against cestodes. Therefore, using such anthelmintic agents in cats will neither protect against nor treat cestode infections. Vigilance must be employed with at-risk patients having a history of access to rodents and no regular tapeworm treatment. It is important that cats undergo annual faecal examination. Where possible, hunting by cats should be discouraged, but for those that do hunt, tapeworm prevention should be considered.

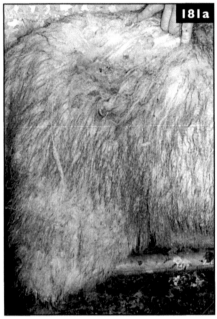

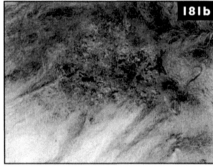

**181** Seventeen sheep that are part of a flock of 70 animals are presented with pruritus, alopecia and crusting, with patches of wool loss particularly prominent over the flanks, dorsum and shoulders. There is also matting and a yellow to brown discolouration of the fleece. Alopecic areas are variably erythematous, excoriated and heavily crusted (**181a, b**). Touching or rubbing lesional areas evokes a 'nibbling' response in most individuals.

i. What is your differential diagnosis for sheep with these clinical signs?
ii. How would you confirm the diagnosis?
iii. How should these sheep be treated?

**181 i.** The large number of animals affected, together with lesion distribution and clinical signs, suggests a highly contagious ectoparasitic infestation, most likely psoroptic mange (scab). Sheep scab should be differentiated from other causes of pruritus, alopecia and crusting in sheep including dermatophilosis (mycotic dermatitis), pediculosis caused by biting (*Damalinia*) or sucking (*Linognathus*) lice species, ked infestation (*Melophagus ovinus*), *Chorioptes* infestation and dermatophytosis.

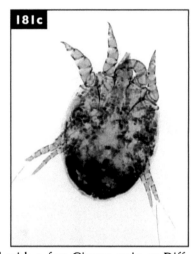

**ii.** Microscopical examination of superficial skin scrapings may reveal numerous *Psoroptes ovis* mites (**181c**), nymphs and eggs. Impression smears can be obtained from the underside of crusts, air-dried and stained with a fast Giemsa stain or Diff-Quik® stain and examined under oil immersion to look for *Dermatophilus* species.

**iii.** The whole flock should be isolated and treated with an effective dip or injectable acaricidal agent. No pour-on, spray or jetting product is effective in the treatment and control of scab. Because of the problems associated with dipping of 70 sheep (labour-intensive procedure with potential chemical dangers to handlers and environment), an injectable acaricidal product is recommended. Ivermectin, although licensed for control of sheep scab when injected twice, 7 days apart, offers little protection against reinfestation. Also sheep must be moved after each treatment to a fresh pasture that has not carried sheep for the previous 16 days. Doramectin requires one injection for treatment and control. Moxidectin, a milbemycin, has been demonstrated in laboratory and field conditions to be highly effective in the treatment of sheep scab. Visibly affected animals should be separated from the flock until the second injection and given supplementary feeding. Trailers and pens should be thoroughly disinfected and no sheep should leave or enter the flock for at least 3 weeks. In addition, newly purshased sheep should be quarantined and treated before entering the flock. These measures should lead to complete resolution.

182 A 4-year-old female alpaca is presented with weight loss of 6–8 weeks' duration. On observation it is noted that she is constantly biting the distal aspects of both forelimbs. Closer inspection reveals that the fleece fibres over the limbs distal to the carpi are broken and the skin is hyperaemic and thickened.

i. What is the differential diagnosis for these clinical signs?

ii. How would you distinguish between these diagnoses?

iii. How would you treat this animal?

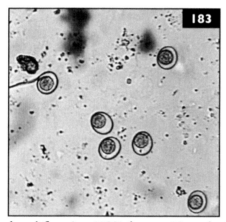

183 You examine a faecal flotation (183) from a 10-week-old captive-bred peregrine falcon displaying signs of lethargy, inappetence and weight loss.

i. Identify this parasite.

ii. Describe its life cycle.

iii. How would you treat this individual?

**182 i.** Sarcoptic mange; chorioptic mange; bacterial folliculitis; dermato–philosis; dermatophytosis; biting and sucking lice; immune-mediated skin disease. The lesion distribution suggests sarcoptic or chorioptic mange, more likely sarcoptic mange because of the degree of pruritus.

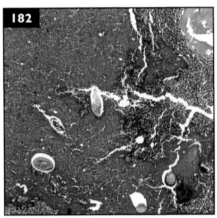

**ii.** With cytology from a deep skin scrape, swab or hair brushing, histopathology from a skin biopsy and culture of a swab from an affected, but non-traumatized, area of the limb. Mites are not always easy to find on scrapes, particularly in the acute phase of disease, which is why multiple samples should be taken from different parts of the limbs. *Sarcoptes scabei* was confirmed on histopathology from a skin biopsy (**182**).

**iii.** Most treatments for sarcoptic mange are not licensed in South American camelids. Treatments include frequent subcutaneous ivermectin, topical eprinomectin, doramectin, selamectin or moxidectin, or a combination of parenteral and topical products. The fibres of alpacas do not contain lanolin, which is necessary for the effective spreading of topically applied products, and this may partly explain therapeutic failures in alpacas. When using pour-ons it is necessary to apply the products directly to the skin. Judicious use of anti-inflammatories may be required in very pruritic individuals. Secondary bacterial infections may require antibiotic treatment.

**183 i.** *Caryospora* species.

**ii.** Adult birds demonstrate a pre-breeding season increase in faecal shedding of oocysts. Oocysts sporulate and become infective 2–4 days after being shed and remain viable in the environment for up to 12 months.

**iii.** Toltrazuril (25 mg/kg PO once weekly for 3 weeks) appears most effective. The 2.5% solution designed for poultry is strongly alkaline and may cause emesis; dilution 50:50 with a carbonated drink may reduce the likelihood of emesis or, alternatively, a 5% solution may be better tolerated. Supportive care with systemic antibiotics, fluid therapy and oral administration of electrolyte solutions and critical care formulas may be required in severe cases.

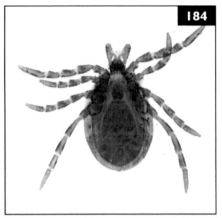

**184** What makes hard ticks (**184**) efficient vectors of diseases?

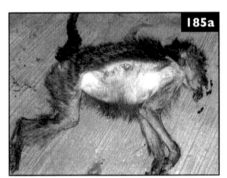

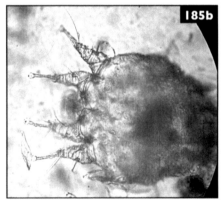

**185** An intensely pruritic baboon of Kenyan origin is presented with extensive alopecia on the abdomen (**185a**). This organism (**185b**) is found on microscopical examination of skin scrapings taken from alopecic areas.
i. What is the organism?
ii. How should this animal be treated?

**184** They are haematophagous ectoparasites and have a remarkable ability to transmit a wide variety of pathogens to humans and animals compared with other arthropods. Ticks can transmit infectious pathogens to the host mechanically when they move from one host to another and their mouthparts are contaminated with blood-containing agents. Ticks can also transmit pathogens biologically, where the pathogen undertakes some sort of development or maturation within the tick. After this occurs, the pathogen is transferred either transstadially (between stages) or transovarially (from female to offspring via the egg).

The important role of ticks in disease transmission is reinforced by the fact that ticks have a worldwide distribution, can adapt to diverse environments and feed for extended periods of time and on a variety of vertebrate hosts as they develop from juveniles to adults. Even one-host ticks, such as *Boophilus* (*Rhipicephalus*) *microplus*, cause major losses to bovine herds, especially in tropical regions. Ticks have a long, slow life cycle that takes several years. Because of this longevity, ticks can carry infectious organisms over prolonged periods of time, thereby not only serving as vectors, but also acting as reservoir hosts for the pathogens they carry. Ticks have salivary glands that play a major role not only in pathogen transmission and establishment, but also in the secretion of bioactive products of various critical functions (e.g. antihaemostatic, anti-inflammatory and immunosuppressive).

**185 i.** A sarcoptic mange mite, which has a worldwide distribution. Sarcoptic mange is rare in non-human primates and appears to be limited to primates maintained in natural or seminatural settings.
**ii.** This baboon was captured alive via chemical immobilization using ketamine (10 mg/kg). Treatment involved the use of ivermectin (0.3 mg/kg SC, repeated after 10 days for 4 weeks). This treatment regimen was sufficient to cause complete resolution of the clinical signs.

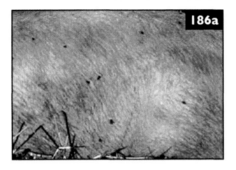

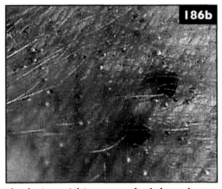

186 Numerous individual pigs within pens of adult and young pigs show rubbing of the flanks and slight pallor and depression. The pigs are housed in an older draughty farm shed, which has housed pigs for many years. Close examination of the pigs reveals several cutaneous parasites on the abdominal flanks (186a), on the proximal aspects of the legs and on the ears. Closer examination of these parasites under a hand lens shows not only adults, but egg-like structures (186b).
i. What is the name of this parasite, and how does it feed on the pig?
ii. What are the small pale egg-like structures?

187 An outbreak of diarrhoeal illness causes the death of 12 guinea pigs at a pet 'superstore'. A diagnosis of coccidiosis is confirmed. Diarrhoea is also noted in rabbits in the same pet shop.
i. What is the name of the parasite that causes intestinal coccidiosis in guinea pigs?
ii. Can the rabbit illness be attributed to the same parasite that is causing the deaths in guinea pigs? Explain.
iii. How can this disease be prevented?

186 i. *Haematopinus suis*, the giant pig louse (186c), which only infests pigs. It grips the hair on the skin with its claws and moves along in a side-to-side fashion. Young nymphs spend much of their time in the ears; as they mature, they move to the abdominal region. Adult *H. suis* are the largest of the sucking lice, measuring >0.5 cm long. They feed exclusively on pig blood; their modified mouthparts burrow into skin venules for feeding. *H. suis* is a permanent parasite; if it becomes dislodged from the host, it only lives for 2 or 3 days, compared with an average 35-day lifespan spent in association with the host.

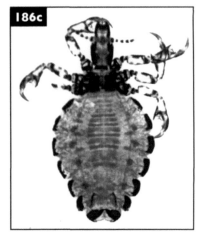

**186c**

ii. The small pale structures are lice eggs ('nits'). After mating, females lay eggs on the pig's hair close to the skin. They lay 3–6 eggs a day for about 25 days. The eggs have an operculum, which serves as lid, cover and flap. It has small holes for gas exchange. Most eggs stay in the local pig environment and hatch in 12–20 days. Female lice provide nutrients to their eggs before laying them, and abandon them afterwards.

187 i. *Eimeria caviae*, a protozoan parasite.
ii. No. The two observations would not have an identical aetiological agent because *Eimeria* species are strictly host specific (the rabbit species cannot infect guinea pigs and vice versa).
iii. Control of *Eimeria* infection in captive situations requires strict attention to sanitation and good husbandry including continual removal of contaminated feed and litter, avoidance of stress and frequent disinfection of cages, hutches, transport carriers and litter pans by steam cleaning, immersion in boiling water or by a 10% ammonia solution ('household' ammonia), which is lethal to coccidial oocysts that are often resistant to many disinfectants. However, if ammonia solution is used, all equipment must be thoroughly rinsed to remove residual solution, which is caustic to mucous membranes and skin.

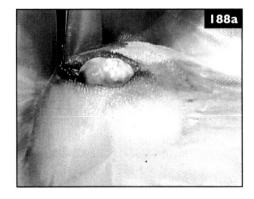

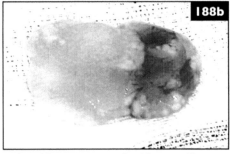

188 A 2-year-old female rabbit is presented with a swelling over the left side of the ribcage. Surgical exploration reveals the presence of a 5-cm diameter cystic mass (188a). The resected cyst has a translucent capsule and contains slightly opaque fluid along with numerous white granules (188b).

i. What is your differential diagnosis?

ii. How would you confirm your diagnosis?

iii. What are the treatment options for this rabbit? Compare the likely effectiveness of the various options.

188 i. Includes abscess, cellulitis, cyst, neoplasm, foreign body granuloma, traumatic haematoma and encysted tapeworm metacestode. The morphological appearance of the resected cyst is suggestive of the cysticercus stage of a tapeworm (188b).

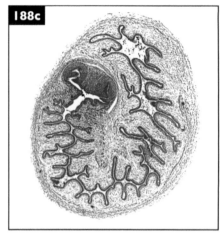

ii. Traditional identification techniques are unhelpful because parasite eggs are not present in the rabbit's faeces. Cytological evaluation of fine needle aspiration will determine the nature of the cyst's content and PCR will confirm the species identity of the cestode. Radiology, CT and MRI should be considered. In this case, histopathological examination showed a cyst containing serous fluid. The multiple dots on the surface of the cyst were protoscolices (188c) of encysted metacestodes. These features are consistent with the larval stage of a *Taenia* species tapeworm, most likely *T. serialis* because the protoscolices are arranged in lines (versus clustered arrangement of protoscolices in *T. multiceps*) and it is the only *Taenia* species known to develop coenurus cysts in subcutaneous tissues and muscles of rabbits.

iii. Medical and surgical interventions have been advocated for treatment of rabbit cysticercosis caused by *T. serialis* coenurus infection. Oral praziquantel and albendazole can be effective. Praziquantel exerts its action by inducing muscle contraction and vacuolization of the cestode's tegument in the growth zone of the neck region, leading to the death of the parasite. Albendazole irreversibly binds tubulin, disrupting cell function, with loss of microtubules and cell death. While effective, death of cestode larvae can lead to a marked inflammatory reaction by the host, which can be ameliorated by concurrent administration of corticosteroids. Coenurus infection can also be managed by surgical excision of the whole coenurus cysts. Leakage of cyst fluid during surgery is unlikely to reseed new cysts and surgery is often curative. Additionally, coenurus cysts can be punctured and the contents aspirated without affecting the rabbit's health.

189 A 4-year-old neutered male dog is presented with anal irritation and rubbing its perineum along the ground. Parasite eggs (189) are observed on faecal flotation.

i. What parasite do you think is causing this dog's signs, and how do you confirm the diagnosis?
ii. How is this parasite transmitted?
iii. What treatment options exist for this infection?
iv. Is this parasite zoonotic?

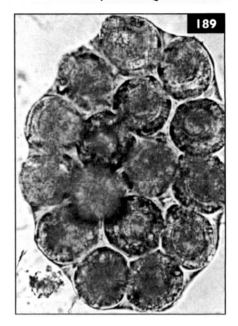

190 A 14-year-old female red-tailed guenon of African origin is presented with a 1-year history of a grossly distended abdomen, leading to distress. Ultrasound examination reveals numerous cystic mass lesions in the abdominal cavity. A lateral abdominal MRI scan is performed (190).

i. What is your differential diagnosis for these clinical signs?
ii. What is the prognosis?
iii. What are the treatment options?
iv. What is the public health implication of this infection?

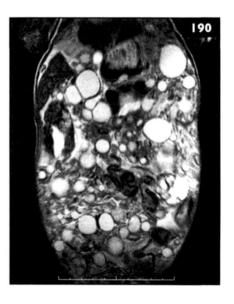

**189 i.** The unique morphology of egg packets of 15–30 eggs in the faeces confirms the diagnosis of the dog tapeworm *Dipylidium caninum*. Proglottids with their 'cucumber seed' shape can be seen crawling on the dog's coat. Segments are usually described as 'rice grain-like', with two common genital pores, one on each margin of each mature segment, which enables differentiation from segments of *Taenia*, which has only one pore.

**ii.** Adult tapeworms reside in the small intestine and gravid proglottids pass out with faeces. They disintegrate and release eggs, which are ingested by the larvae of an IH such as the flea (*Ctenocephalides* species) dog louse (*Trichodectes canis*) or human flea (*Pulex irritans*). The tapeworm matures into a cysticercoid stage in the developing fleas or lice. Dogs become infected after ingestion of an infected IH. Cysticercoid larvae are then released and grow to maturity in the dog's intestine about 1 month after infection.

**iii.** Treatment of choice is praziquantel (niclosamide and epsiprantel are also effective) combined with measures to control fleas and lice to limit the opportunity for dogs to acquire infection through ingestion of infected fleas or lice. Because flea infestation is difficult to prevent entirely, routine monthly deworming of some dogs may be indicated.

**iv.** Yes. Humans can accidentally ingest an infected flea or louse.

**190 i.** Includes abdominal hydatidosis, abdominal abscess, cysticercosis, hepatic carcinoma, hepatic abscesses, hepatic cysts, tuberculosis, biliary cirrhosis, right-sided heart disease and peritonitis. Based on the MRI scan and the disseminated pattern of the lesions, abdominal hydatidosis caused by *Echinococcus* species infection is the most likely cause in this animal.

**ii.** Very poor. The disseminated infection and wide distribution pattern of the hydatid cysts in this animal indicate that some underlying immunosuppressive disease exists, which allowed for this extensive degree of parasite infection. This pattern could also be due to multiple infections, a genetically susceptible host or prior rupture of a cyst. Aggressive treatment is necessary. Even then, there is no guarantee of survival.

**iii.** Albendazole and mebendazole have been used with limited success. In this case, treatment is at best palliative and may simply extend the lifespan of the affected monkey.

**iv.** Hydatid infection poses public health risks in that guenon to carnivore and, possibly, carnivore to human transmission of hydatidosis could create a perpetual reservoir of complicated infections. It is critical that the carcass of the dead animal is disposed of hygienically (e.g. incineration) and in such a way that does not allow canids access.

**191** A 3-year-old female Pit Bull Terrier from Texas (USA) is presented for evaluation after a 3-day history of progressive lethargy, icteric mucous membranes, weakness and anorexia. A stained blood smear is made (**191**).

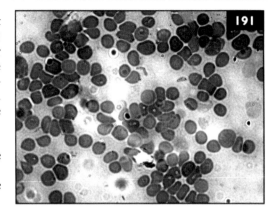

i. What is your diagnosis?
ii. How did the dog become infected with this parasite?
iii. How should this case be managed?

**192 i.** Match the following pesticide agent with its mechanism of action:

| a. | Fipronil | 1. | An agonist to nicotinic acetylcholine receptors in post-synaptic nerve membranes. |
|---|---|---|---|
| b. | Imidacloprid | 2. | Increases permability in neuronal chloride channels. This increase in permeability and rapid influx of chloride ions inhibit the electric activity of target insects and result in rapid flaccid paralysis with death and elimination from the host. |
| c. | Nitenpyram | 3. | Acts on the GABA receptor as a non-competitive blocker of the GABA-gated chloride channels or glutamate-gated channels. Blockade of the GABA receptors results in neural excitation and death in target insects. |
| d. | Selamectin | 4. | Disrupts the synthesis and deposition of chitin of target insects by blocking the enzyme chitin synthetase. It has no deleterious effects on the adult fleas, but has ovicidal and larvicidal activity. |
| e. | Lufenuron | 5. | Binds to nicotinergic receptors in post-synaptic nerves to prevent acetylcholine from binding and transmitting information. Receptor blockade results in impairment of normal nerve function and death of the insect. |

ii. What are the common causes of insecticide resistance?
iii. List some general strategies or recommendations for when using insecticides.

**191 i.** Infection with *Babesia gibsoni*, a haemoprotozoan parasite. Microscopically, the parasite forms small, round to oval piroplasms measuring 1.0–2.5 μm in diameter.
**ii.** Following attachment of an infected tick, *Babesia* sporozoites are released into the blood, infecting erythrocytes. Binary fission (an asexual form of division) occurs in the cytoplasm of the RBC and results in merozoites. Ticks become infected with merozoites during feeding and can remain infective for more than one generation via transovarial and transstadial transmission. *B. gibsoni* is also transmitted by direct blood contamination; potential sources include dog fights and sharing of surgical instruments. Transplacental transmission from bitch to offspring can also occur.
**iii.** With a combination of atovaquone (13.3 mg/kg q8h) and azithromycin (10 mg/kg q24h). Glucocorticoids can be used at acute stages to reduce immune-mediated RBC destruction; however, long-term use may result in decreased splenic clearance of the organism. Two injections of imidocarb dipropionate (5.0–6.6 mg/kg SC or IM at an interval of 2–3 weeks) are effective. Supportive therapy such as intravenous fluids and blood transfusions should be employed when necessary. Prevention of *B. gibsoni* infection includes tick control, sterilizing surgical instruments, screening programmes in breeding kennels and prevention of dog fighting. Animals that survive babesiosis remain subclinically infected and these dogs may suffer a relapse of disease in the future or serve as point sources for further spread of disease.

**192 i.** (a – 3); (b – 5); (c – 1); (d – 2); (e – 4).
**ii.** The loss of efficacy of insecticides can be attributed to (1) diminished penetration into the target organism, (2) increased detoxication (metabolism) of insecticides, (3) decreased sensitivity of the target site (i.e. receptor) or (4) increased excretion via P-glycoprotein-related pumps.
**iii.** Reduce the number of treatments and use insecticides only when necessary. Consider reducing dependence on insecticides and integrate procedures for managing animal ectoparasites to avoid promoting resistance to currently effective agents. Continuously monitor for the presence of resistance to optimize the timing of insecticide use and to determine the need for additional treatments. Administer the insecticide effectively (always follow the manufacturer's instructions). Avoid introducing resistant insects – use quarantine treatments. Adopt strategies to maintain refugia (i.e. susceptible individuals) which, by mating with resistant individuals, reduces the resistance level of the population.

**193** You are presented in early summer with two 3-year-old castrated male reindeer that are depressed and have reduced appetites; one also has diarrhoea. These are part of a herd of 10 reindeer that live in a 2-acre enclosure that is partially concrete and partially grass; the grass is very short. There is no paddock rotation. The reindeer are fed commercial goat pellets and hay. They are not vaccinated and were last dewormed with injectable doramectin 12 months ago. One reindeer from this herd died 5 days ago after showing similar clinical signs for 2 days. Gross post-mortem examination reveals no abnormalities. The worm egg count from the faeces of this reindeer at the time of its death was 1,500 epg (trichostrongyle eggs).
**i.** What are the potential management problems with these reindeer? Compare this with their behaviour in their natural habitat.
**ii.** What clinical presentations are seen in ruminants with trichostrongyle infection?
**iii.** How would you manage and treat these affected individuals and the in-contacts in this group?

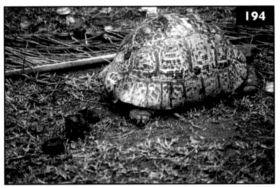

**194** A captive tortoise defecates (**194**).
**i.** Which species of tortoise is this?
**ii.** List the parasites that might be detected in the faeces.
**iii.** Are any of zoonotic potential?
**iv.** Should such parasites be routinely treated?

**193 i.** Reindeer are browsers and rarely eat grass. They also travel over large distances so are unaccustomed to ingestion of faecal parasites. As they originate from relatively cold climates, the period when infective larvae are available for ingestion would also be short. These reindeer live in a small paddock with a high stocking density and were last dewormed 12 months ago. Since effective removal of the small faecal pellets from the grass part of the paddock is impractical, the worm burden in this area will remain high, particularly in a temperate climate during the summer. Reindeer are easier to manage in small spaces when they are kept on concrete, which can be easily cleaned.
**ii.** Trichostrongylosis is often associated with non-specific signs including poor production, unthriftiness, diarrhoea and weight loss. Unless infection is severe, disease in ruminants would not normally be as severe as in this instance, particularly with a presumed mild to moderate infection.
**iii.** Management includes supportive care for the diarrhoea and depression and eradication of the parasites in affected and in-contact animals. Affected reindeer were treated with parenteral corticosteroids and NSAIDs to combat intestinal inflammation and systemic inflammatory responses secondary to bacteraemia. They were also treated with parenteral antimicrobials because of the likelihood of secondary bacteraemia. All were treated with parenteral ivermectin. Reindeer may not respond appropriately to injectable doramectin. Ideally, animals need to rotate through multiple paddocks. If this is not possible, a concrete pen allows for more effective parasite control. Feeding off the ground will reduce the number of eggs ingested. A prophylactic anthelmintic protocol should be instituted to prevent development of clinical disease in the future.

**194 i.** A leopard tortoise, which is found throughout sub-Saharan Africa. Large numbers of this species are now kept in captivity, often successfully bred, in Europe and North America.
**ii.** Various protozoa, nematodes and trematodes.
**iii.** They are unlikely to be zoonotic. However, ascarids and oxyurids have direct life cycles with autoinfection, and parasite populations can quickly build up in the immediate environment. Also, bacterial infection, especially salmonellosis, is a recognized danger from these and some other reptiles.
**iv.** Treatment may be desirable in captivity. Whenever possible, treatment should follow the examination of faeces for evidence of parasites. Work on Mediterranean tortoises suggests that certain nematodes that live in the large intestine may in fact be beneficial because they help to break down plant material and make it available for digestion by commensal protozoa and bacteria.

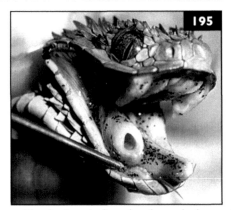

**195** A recently captured bush viper is found to have dark, particulate bodies in its buccal cavity (**195**).
**i.** What are these bodies?
**ii.** How might these structures be best removed for identification?

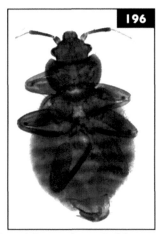

**196** This pest (**196**) is collected from a household in a rural village.
**i.** What is it, and how does it feed?
**ii.** Describe its typical environment and clinical significance.
**iii.** What are the treatment options in humans?
**iv.** How would you control this pest?

**195 i.** Trematodes of the genus *Mesocoelium*. They are parasites of amphibians and lizards and largely confined to Africa. The larvae are found in molluscs, which are the IHs. The adult flukes are usually located in the intestine of the reptile, but occasionally, as in this case, they migrate through the stomach, up through the oesophagus and into the buccal cavity. The fluke feeds on food debris and mucus in the gastrointestinal tract of the reptile.
**ii.** By using a cotton bud soaked in normal saline. They can then be mounted for microscopical examination.

**196 i.** The bed bug *Cimex lectularius*, a wingless insect 5–7 mm in length. Bed bugs are obligate blood-feeding ectoparasites of humans and other warm-blooded animals. They usually become active at night and prefer feeding when host activity is minimal.
**ii.** After a meal, they leave the host and retire to a safe haven (e.g. in cracks, under mattresses or in other dark places), where they survive for months without feeding. Although bed bugs are not likely to act as vectors of diseases, they cause loss of sleep, general discomfort, psychological distress and unpleasant skin irritation due to their blood-feeding behaviour. Some individuals are sensitive to bed bug bites and show allergic reactions. Affected areas are usually those exposed while sleeping. Bed bug infestation imposes economic loss on the household owing to the costs of pest control and replacement of infested infrastructure.
**iii.** Reducing pruritus with topical corticosteroids and oral antihistamines and preventing secondary bacterial infection due to scratching and excoriation. Secondary infection is treated with topical or systemic antibiotics.
**iv.** By thorough inspection of the infested sites and application of insecticides such as pyrethroids. However, insecticide resistance has been reported with increasing frequency and is a likely reason for the recent bed bug resurgence in developed countries. Severely infested mattresses should be discarded. Early detection may help retard spread into non-infested areas.

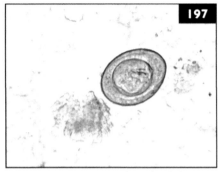

**197** A 2-year-old male pet rat is presented with abdominal pain and diarrhoea associated with weight loss and reduced appetite. This parasite egg (**197**) was seen microscopically in a fresh faecal smear.

**i.** What is this egg?
**ii.** Describe its life cycle.
**iii.** Is this parasite zoonotic?
**iv.** How can this infection be treated and prevented?

**198** Several diurnal and nocturnal birds of prey hospitalized in a raptor rehabilitation centre appear ruffled and emaciated, with signs of laboured breathing. Some of them have large masses around the oropharynx (**198**). Some birds died because of anorexia and subsequent starvation. Post-mortem findings revealed large yellowish caseous lesions in the upper digestive and respiratory tract mainly located on the oropharynx, tongue, nasal cavity, hard palate, trachea and larynx. All the birds are fed with fresh pigeons.

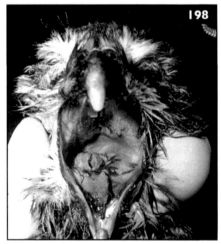

**i.** What is your most likely diagnosis?
**ii.** What is your differential diagnosis?
**iii.** How can you stop the spread of the infection in the raptor centre?
**iv.** How can you treat sick raptors?

197 i. The rat tapeworm *Hymenolepis diminuta*.

ii. *H. diminuta* is a rodent parasite for which coprophilic arthropods (fleas and coleoptera) act as IHs. Rodents, particularly rats, are the definitive hosts and natural reservoirs of *H. diminuta*. Tapeworm eggs ingested by the arthropods develop into cysticercoid larvae within these insects. Rats become infected by ingesting infected insects. The cysticercoids present in the body cavity of the insects break open and develop into adult worms in the rat intestine. The eggs are then passed in the faeces.

iii. Humans, usually children, can accidentally be infected through the same mechanism of ingesting infected fleas. Although uncommon, *H. diminuta* infection in humans has been reported, especially in rural areas. The human intestinal form of *H. diminuta* infection is often asymptomatic, but abdominal pain, irritability, itching and eosinophilia have been reported.

iv. Praziquantel is the drug of choice. Disposal of the bedding hygienically and replacement with clean material is important to prevent the spread of the tapeworm eggs, with cleaning and sterilization or replacement of the rat cage. Control of intermediate insect hosts can assist in breaking the life cycle of tapeworm transmission.

198 i. Trichomonosis (frounce), caused by *Trichomonas gallinae*.

ii. Includes infection by *Aspergillus* species, *Candida* species and nematodes of the genus *Capillaria*, and vitamin A deficiency. Isolation of motile *Trichomonas* stages from fresh saliva or smears made from the caseous lesions is required to confirm *Trichomonas* infection.

iii. Birds of prey are sensitive to *Trichomonas* and transmission occurs through direct contact or ingestion of contaminated food or water. Live pigeons and doves are frequent sources of infection for captive raptors. It has been reported that 80–90% of pigeons and doves are infected, with a high prevalence of asymptomatic carriers. Before pigeons and doves are fed to raptors they should be inspected and their carcasses frozen for at least 24 hours. This procedure appears to kill the parasite or at least significantly reduces its pathogenicity.

iv. Infected birds should be isolated and treated. The drugs of choice are metronidazole and dimetridazole, although ronidazole or carnidazole can be used. Several antiprotozoal agents used in avian medicine have a low therapeutic index and are toxic for certain avian species. (Refer to an avian/exotic animal formulary before starting any treatment.)

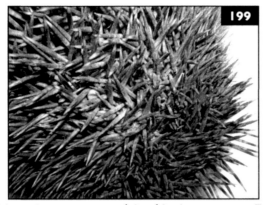

199 This small insectivorous mammal is ubiquitous among European wildlife (199).
i. What is this animal?
ii. Identify the ectoparasite present.
iii. What is the suggested treatment for this parasitic infestation?
iv. Describe the public health risk posed by this animal.

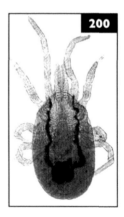

200 Four grower chickens are found dead in a free-range poultry farm. All the carcasses are very pale and large numbers of mites (200) are present in the feathers.
i. What is your diagnosis?
ii. What animal health and welfare issues may be associated with this condition?
iii. How should affected birds be treated?

199 i. A European hedgehog (*Erinaceus europaeus*).
ii. Likely *Ixodes ricinus* (sheep tick, pasture tick, castor bean tick, deer tick), a tick found all over Europe, North Africa and the Middle East. It feeds on numerous different hosts including small mammals, birds and reptiles. It might also be *I. hexagonus*, the hedgehog tick, which is very similar and with similar distribution.
iii. Physical removal of ticks with a proper tick removal device, followed by application of a pyrethroid powder/bath treatment to prevent new infestation.
iv. Injured hedgehogs must be treated as soon as they are hospitalized to avoid environmental contamination of the facilities by ticks. *I. ricinus* can transmit a great number of tick-borne diseases to its hosts, including humans.

200 i. Infestation with the poultry red mite *Dermanyssus gallinae*.
ii. *D. gallinae* infestation may have a serious impact on the production and welfare of laying hens. In high-intensity infestation the mites cause anaemia and even death of infested hens. In moderate to severe infestations, feeding mites may result in significant stress to hens with a resulting negative impact on bird condition, growth rate and egg production. Low-level infestation may pose fewer problems to the birds; however, the mite can serve as a vector for a number of poultry pathogens.
iii. Control has usually been achieved by use of synthetic contact acaricides including carbaryl, diazinon, dichlorvos and permethrin, but the continued use of these products is hampered by issues of mite resistance and decreasing product availability. A recent study has shown that effective control of *D. gallinae* can be achieved for a period of at least 28 days after spraying of spinosad. Treatment with carbaryl dusting powder, or oral ivermectin or moxidectin, is also effective. It is essential to treat the environment at the same time with safe residual insecticides. Neem tree oil has been used successfully for red mite control.

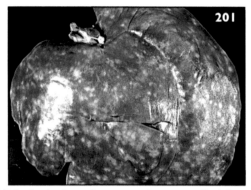

**201** A well-established pig farm has several open-walled but sheltered grower–finisher pens. The farmer uses deep straw bedding over a soil base within the pens. The abattoir regularly reports back to the farmer regarding lesions (**201**) in the livers of slaughtered pigs.

**i.** What are these lesions, and how are they formed?

**ii.** What clinical significance does this hold?

**iii.** What other conditions would you want to check for on this farm that may be part of an enteric complex?

**202** A 2-year-old male bearded dragon is found dead. On necropsy, the liver appears yellow and spotted. Histologically, the yellow foci correspond to areas of inflammation with many scattered organisms (**202**).

**i.** What organisms are most likely present in these lesions?

**ii.** How would you confirm your diagnosis?

**iii.** What advice would you give to the owner?

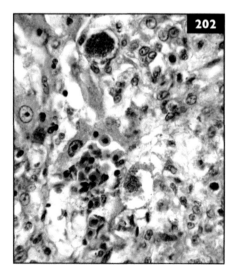

**201 i.** Whitish healing foci ('milk spots'), which occur in the liver stroma when migrating *Ascaris suum* larvae are immobilized by the host's inflammatory reaction. Milk spot lesions observed in the abattoir generally provide information on *A. suum* challenge in the last 4 weeks before slaughter.

**ii.** The presence of milk spots leads to considerable losses due to offal condemnations. Housing conditions (i.e. floor type) and management practices (e.g. cleaning and disinfection procedures; type of feeding) play an important role in the development of *A. suum*. Milk spots, if present, tend to occur asymptomatically, being incidental post-mortem findings. Therefore, the presence of *A. suum*, or its lesions, cannot easily be detected in the live pig. Diagnosis is made either directly (faecal egg detection or serology) or indirectly (presence of migration lesions in lung or milk spots in liver).

**iii.** Besides nematode parasitism, other oral–faecal transmitted diseases will thrive in bedding or outdoor systems where the floor cannot be cleaned. In some cases, pigs will suffer an enteric disease complex consisting of ileitis due to *Lawsonia intracellularis*, colitis due to *Brachyspira* species, salmonellosis and ascariosis. Although not really an enteric disease, experience suggests that erysipelas is also common in these systems, due to oral infection derived from soil and bedding contamination. The potential rise of salmonellosis in particular under these systems raises food safety concerns.

**202 i.** The morphological features of the organisms contained within the rounded vacuoles suggest infection with an apicomplexan protozoan parasite, such as *Toxoplasma gondii* or *Neospora caninum*.

**ii.** By immunohistochemistry. However, because of the possibility of false-positive results due to serological cross-reactivity, further testing (e.g. electron microcsopic characterization and/or genetic analysis using PCR) is essential to confirm the diagnosis (*T. gondii* in this case).

**iii.** Cats and other felids are the only known definitive hosts for *T. gondii*. Infection in the bearded dragon was probably associated with ingestion of oocysts excreted in the faeces of cats. Scavenging on infected rats is another possible route of infection. Therefore, to prevent occurrence of the same infection in the future, cats should not be allowed to have contact with bearded dragons. Owners should also be aware of the high zoonotic potential of *T. gondii*, especially for pregnant women and immunocompromised individuals.

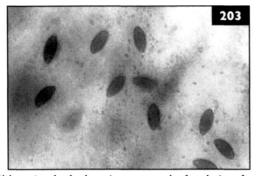

203 A young, wild native hedgehog is presented after being found wandering in a residential area in the middle of the day. The hedgehog appears underweight, tachypnoeic and dyspnoeic and has green diarrhoea. A microscopic image of a fresh faecal smear is shown (203).
i. What are the objects on the smear?
ii. Would they explain the clinical signs described?
iii. How would you treat this patient?

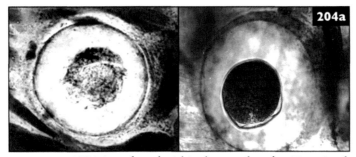

204 These structures (204a) are found within the muscles of an Egyptian freshwater tilapian fish.
i. What are they?
ii. What is their significance?

**203 i.** *Capillaria* species eggs. Hedgehogs are host to several species of *Capillaria*; *C. aerophila* affects the lungs, *C. erinacei* and *C. ovoreticulata* affect the intestines.
**ii.** *Capillaria* infection is often asymptomatic, but heavy burdens may cause respiratory signs (*C. aerophila*) or green, mucoid diarrhoea and weight loss (*C. erinacei* and *C. ovoreticulata*). Mixed lung infections with *Crenosoma striatum* are common and may exacerbate respiratory signs and predispose to secondary bacterial infections.
**iii.** Levamisole and fenbendazole are effective anthelmintics in the hedgehog. Supportive care, including oxygen therapy, nebulization, mucolytics and systemic antibiotics, may be required depending on the severity of the clinical signs.

**204 i.** Encysted metacercaria (larval stage) of digenetic trematodes. The dimensions of these metacercariae (cyst size, 260–340 µm; cyst wall thickness, 5.5–9.2 µm) are consistent with those of the family Heterophyidae, a group of minute intestinal trematodes infecting avian and mammalian hosts. The larval stage encysts in the muscles of fish, whereas adult flukes inhabit the intestines of fish-eating mammals, including humans. Species identity can be confirmed via the morphological characteristics of adult flukes (**204b**) recovered from small intestines of laboratory-reared, parasite-free puppies approximately 3 weeks after feeding the puppies with the metacercaria.
**ii.** Freshwater fish are IHs and a source of human infection for many heterophyid trematodes. More than 22 heterophyid species that cycle in marine or freshwater fish are known to infect humans worldwide. Human infections are usually mild. However, infection with heterophyids can be accompanied by abdominal pain and diarrhoea, and the parasite egg can disseminate haematogenously to extra-intestinal locations and may produce eosinophilic granulomas in the heart, brain and spinal cord (in both humans and animals).

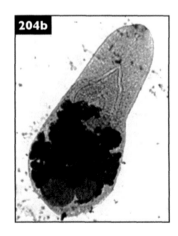

205 Data in the table below represent faecal egg counts (FECs) carried out using the McMaster technique on faecal samples from 15 randomly selected sheep 1 week before and 2 weeks after treatment with fenbendazole. The FEC reduction (FECR) for each animal has been calculated using the formula below:

$$\text{FECR (\%)} = 100 \times \left[ 1 - \frac{\text{mean FEC after treatment}}{\text{mean FEC before treatment}} \right]$$

| Sheep No. | FEC (before treatment) | FEC (after treatment) | FECR (%) |
|---|---|---|---|
| 1 | 250 | 50 | 80 |
| 2 | 1,369 | 0 | 100 |
| 3 | 960 | 0 | 100 |
| 4 | 0 | 0 | 0 |
| 5 | 3,450 | 150 | 95.6 |
| 6 | 1,900 | 0 | 100 |
| 7 | 1,389 | 317 | 77.1 |
| 8 | 2,400 | 45 | 98.1 |
| 9 | 0 | 0 | 0 |
| 10 | 1,250 | 0 | 100 |
| 11 | 1,190 | 0 | 100 |
| 12 | 0 | 0 | 0 |
| 13 | 2,200 | 25 | 98.8 |
| 14 | 1,960 | 45 | 97.7 |
| 15 | 640 | 0 | 100 |
| | 1,263.86 | 42.13 | 96.6 |

i. Considering a good anthelmintic efficacy is defined as FECR ≥95%, is there any indication that there are nematodes resistant to fendendazole on the farm?
ii. What measures should be taken to slow down the development of resistance to fendendazole on this farm?

206 A 5-year-old spider monkey at a zoo presents with diarrhoea of 3 days duration. Faecal investigation reveals this organism (206).
i. What is present in the faeces?
ii. How can infection by this parasite be managed?

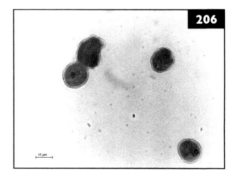

**205 i.** The average for the flock is 1,263.86 ± 1,006 before treatment and 42.13 ± 85.9 after treatment, giving an overall FECR of 96.6%. On a flock level there does not appear to be a problem with using fenbendazole. However, at the individual level, two sheep (1 and 7) have an FECR of <95%. This indicates that worms in these two sheep are less susceptible to fenbendazole and that there is a potential for resistance to this drug to develop in the flock; however, this apparent prevalence of reduced anthelmintic efficacy may not necessarily be attributed to the presence of resistant parasites, but could also be due to other confounding factors such as the incorrect administration of the anthelmintic or underdosing of the two sheep.
**ii.** Treat only those sheep that need therapy. The rest of the flock should be left untreated as a reservoir of unselected worms. This will dilute out the worms in which resistance to the drug has been selected for. Breed only from sheep that have shown a natural resistance to GI parasitic nematodes and eventually a flock will develop that needs little anthelmintic treatment. Resistance to fenbendazole is so widespread that it should be used with caution in prophylactic dosing regimens unless FECR proves that the drug is still effective.

**206 i.** Trophozoites of *Entamoeba* species.
**ii.** Treat affected animals with an amoebicidal drug such as metronidazole. *Entamoeba* infection is a significant zoonotic disease in non-human primates, therefore good hygiene, sanitation and husbandry practices are critical in reducing *Entamoeba* infection risks as they disturb the faecal–oral route of transmission. Quarantine procedures for new arrivals should include faecal examination on multiple samples utilizing the most accurate detection method available. Important precautionary measures include hygienic food preparation with good quality water, appropriate hand disinfection and disinfection or disposal of keeper footwear, clothing and gloves and enclosure cleaning equipment. Disinfection must be practised when moving between different animal enclosures. Microfiltration of water features within enclosures and effective drainage within and between enclosures is critical. Proactive pest control reduces arthropod vectors, including houseflies and cockroaches, which can transport the infective cystic stage between enclosures.

207 A 6-day-old Holstein male calf is presented with a 2-day history of anorexia, lethargy and haemorrhagic diarrhoea (207). Despite the use of antibiotics, fluid therapy and supportive care, the calf dies within 12 hours. You suspect *Cryptosporidium* infection.

**i.** What husbandry practices contribute to this infection?
**ii.** What are the available treatment options?
**iii.** How would you prevent this problem?

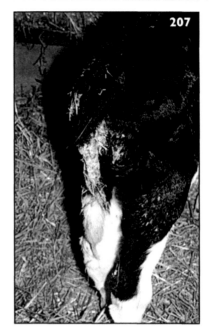

208 A 5-year-old Thorough-bred horse has recently been purchased with no known history and moved to a small property with four other horses. The horse is showing clinical signs of moderate to

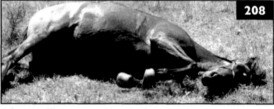

severe abdominal pain (208), such as rolling, sweating, kicking at its abdomen and flank watching. Physical examination reveals dark oral pink mucous membranes, capillary refill time of 3 seconds and poor pulse quality. Heart rate is 68 beats per minute and borborygmi are absent in all four quadrants. Rectal examination reveals no obvious abnormalities, although the horse is uncomfortable on palpation of the intestines. Nasogastric intubation recovers no fluid, but peritoneocentesis recovers serosanguineous fluid with a total solids of 30 g/l (normal <20 g/l).

**i.** What is your differential diagnosis for this case, and what parasitic diseases in particular should be considered?
**ii.** What would you recommend regarding management of this case?

**207 i.** Inadequate management measures, including intensive dairy cattle production, overcrowding, poor hygiene and direct contact between animals, are risk factors for cryptosporidiosis and other diarrhoeal diseases on farms.

**ii.** There is no specific antiparasitic chemotherapy for cryptosporidiosis. Most immunocompetent animals recover within 1–2 weeks of infection with supportive care (e.g. fluid therapy). Paromycin has been used with limited success in cats and human patients, but its efficacy in other species has not been determined. Oral bovine serum concentrate has been used in calves with experimentally induced cryptosporidiosis. Bovine serum administration reduces the volume of diarrhoea, reduces intestinal permeability and enhances ideal crypt depth and villous surface area (i.e. promotes epithelial regeneration). There are no vaccines approved for prevention of bovine cryptosporidiosis.

**iii.** *Cryptosporidium* species are highly zoonotic. Any contact with affected animals will lead to infection, therefore better management of cryptosporidiosis is essential from both veterinary and public health points of view. Good hygiene is important in reducing the incidence of infection transmission. Measures include cleaning maternity pens, housing and feeding equipment and isolating sick calves to a separate area to reduce contamination, plus early detection of anorexia, diarrhoea and dehydration in neonatal calves. Dam and calf should be provided with good nutrition. Administration of high-quality colostrum within the first 6 hours after birth helps reduce infection. Halofuginone is approved for use against calf cryptosporidiosis.

**208 i.** Possible differential diagnoses include a small intestinal strangulating lipoma and epiploic foramen entrapment of a loop of small intestine. The latter would be more likely due to the lack of increased fluid obtained on nasogastric intubation and no distended loops of small intestine palpable on rectal examination. The horse could also have a large colonic volvulus, although it would be expected to be in more pain and have more severe abnormalities on clinical evaluation. Other possibilities include colitis or enterocolitis that has not yet produced diarrhoea. Possible aetiologies for this include emergence of cyathostome larvae with recent anthelmintic treatment, right dorsal colitis secondary to NSAID administration and infectious causes (e.g. *Clostridium* species, *Salmonella* species and *Neorickettsia risticii* [Potomac horse fever]). Ischaemic damage to the intestine caused by thrombi formation can also cause this presentation, the most common cause being the migrating larval stages (L4) of *Strongylus vulgaris*.

**ii.** Analgesia and sedation could be provided, but a poor prognosis should be anticipated. On referral to a surgical centre, transabdominal and rectal ultrasound revealed no distended loops of small intestine and no fluid-filled colon. However, the intestinal wall of the left ventral colon was thickened and appeared oedematous. Exploratory laparotomy revealed 1.8 metres of large intestine (including caecum and left ventral colon), which was red to purple in colour. The horse was euthanized and adult *Strongylus vulgaris* worms were found in the caecum and colon.

# Further reading

Bowman DD (2009) *Georgi's Parasitology for Veterinarians*, 9th edn. Elsevier, St Louis.

Colwell DD, Dantas-Torres F, Otranto D (2011) Vector-borne parasitic zoonoses: emerging scenarios and new perspectives. *Vet Parasitol* 182:14–21.

Conboy G (2009) Helminth parasites of the canine and feline respiratory tract. *Vet Clin North Am Small Anim Pract* 39:1109–1126.

Elsheikha HM, Naveed Khan (2011) *Essentials of Veterinary Parasitology*, 1st edn. Caister Academic Press, Wymondham.

Foster N, Elsheikha HM (2012) The immune response to parasitic helminths of veterinary importance and its potential manipulation for future vaccine control strategies. *Parasitol Res* 110:1587–1599.

Francesconi F, Lupi O (2012) Myiasis. *Clin Microbiol Rev* 25:79–105.

Hoste H, Torres-Acosta JF (2011) Non chemical control of helminths in ruminants: adapting solutions for changing worms in a changing world. *Vet Parasitol* 180:144–154.

Nielsen MK, Fritzen B, Duncan JL *et al.* (2010) Practical aspects of equine parasite control: a review based upon a workshop discussion consensus. *Equine Vet J* 42:460–468.

Rivero A, Vézilier J, Weill M *et al.* (2010) Insecticide control of vector-borne diseases: when is insecticide resistance a problem? *PLoS Pathogens* 6(8):e1001000.

Sargison ND (2011) Pharmaceutical control of endoparasitic helminth infections in sheep. *Vet Clin North Am Food Anim Pract* 27:139–156.

Sutherland IA, Leathwick DM (2011) Anthelmintic resistance in nematode parasites of cattle: a global issue? *Trends Parasitol* 27:176–181.

Taylor MA, Coop RL, Wall RL (2007) *Veterinary Parasitology*, 3rd edn. Wiley- Blackwell, Oxford.

Torgerson PR, Macpherson CN (2011) The socioeconomic burden of parasitic zoonoses: global trends. *Vet Parasitol* 182:79–95.

Wall R, Rose H, Ellse L *et al.* (2011) Livestock ectoparasites: integrated management in a changing climate. *Vet Parasitol* 180:82–89.

Wells B, Burgess ST, McNeilly TN *et al.* (2012) Recent developments in the diagnosis of ectoparasite infections and disease through a better understanding of parasite biology and host responses. *Mol Cell Probe* 26:47–53.

Zajac AM, Conboy GA (2006) *Veterinary Clinical Parasitology*, 7th edn. Wiley-Blackwell, Ames.

# Appendix: Life cycles

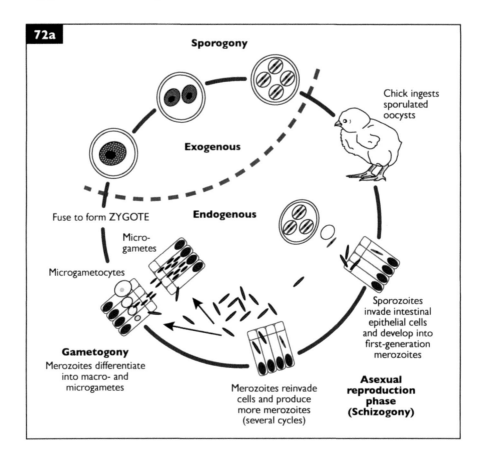

**83**

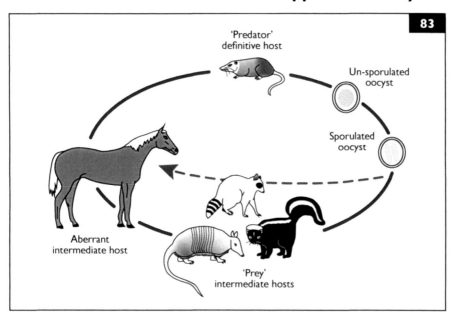

'Predator'
definitive host

Un-sporulated
oocyst

Sporulated
oocyst

Aberrant
intermediate host

'Prey'
intermediate hosts

---

**147c**

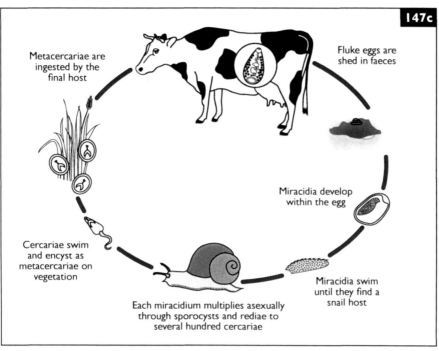

Metacercariae are
ingested by the
final host

Fluke eggs are
shed in faeces

Miracidia develop
within the egg

Cercariae swim
and encyst as
metacercariae on
vegetation

Each miracidium multiplies asexually
through sporocysts and rediae to
several hundred cercariae

Miracidia swim
until they find a
snail host

# Glossary

**Acaricides:** compounds that act against ectoparasites belonging to the Acari group (mites and ticks).

**Anthelmintic:** chemical drug used to remove worms, usually from the intestinal tract and/or respiratory tract of a host.

**Asexual reproduction:** multiplication of parasite stages by binary or multicellular fission without production of sexually differentiated stages.

**Bots:** larvae of several fly species, particularly *Gastrophilus* (horse bot), *Oestrus* (sheep bot) and *Dermatobia* and *Hypoderma* (affect cattle and other species).

**Bradyzoite:** slow-growing zoite or meront of the pseudocyst of *Toxoplasma* and related tissue cyst-forming coccidian protozoa.

**Buccal capsule:** mouth cavity of a nematode.

**Bursa (copulatory bursa):** cuticular copulatory structure at the posterior end of males of the suborder Strongylida. Its morphological attributes are useful in nematode taxonomy and species identification.

**Cercaria (-iae):** free–living larval trematode that develops from a sporocyst or redia in snail intermediate hosts.

**Coenurus:** fluid-filled metacestode of some tapeworms of the family Taeniidae. Has a non-laminated wall that produces protoscolices, but without brood capsules.

**Coprophagous:** feeding on manure.

**Cysticercoid:** tapeworm larva that develops in an invertebrate intermediate host; characteristic of many cyclophyllidean families such as Hymenolepididae, Dilepididae or Anoplocephalidae.

**Cysticercus:** tapeworm larva in which the scolex develops in an inverted form and which has a fluid-filled bladder surrounding it. It is characteristic of the cyclophyllidean family Taeniidae.

**Definitive or final host:** host in which the parasite attains its sexual maturity (cf. intermediate hosts).

**Ectoparasiticide:** compound developed for on-animal use as a therapeutic agent to eliminate any existing ectoparasite infestation and prevent reinfestation.

**Egg or ovum:** germ cell of a female.

**Engorgement:** distension of a feeding tick with blood; cannot occur in male hard ticks because their back is covered completely by a hard scutum.

**Epimeres (= apodemes):** grooves in the cuticle that extend from the base of each leg. Have a diagnostic value in discriminating mites.

**Erratic parasites:** found in their normal hosts, but in unusual organs or tissues in which they are not adapted to live.

**Excystation:** escape of parasite stages from the multilayered shell, which covers the cystic stages, such as oocyst.

**Feral:** feral cycle of a parasitic agent is one that takes place in the wild as opposed to an urban site.

**Gamogony (= gametogony):** formation of gametes.

**Haematophagous:** bloodsucking; usually refers to the feeding habits of various insects and acarines such as mosquitoes and ticks.

**Hexacanth:** six-hooked, first-stage larva of certain tapeworms; stage that hatches from the cestode egg and infects the intermediate host.

**Horizontal transmission:** transmission of a parasitic agent among members of a group.

**Insecticides:** compounds that act against ectoparasites belonging to the Class Insecta.

**Intermediate host:** host that provides the parasite with a temporary environment for completion of immature stages of its life cycle, but one in which only the asexual or immature stages of the parasite occur.

**Juvenile:** organism similar to the adult of the species, but sexually immature.

**Larva:** embryo that becomes self-sustaining and independent before it has developed the characteristic features of the adult form.

**Merogony:** type of asexual reproduction in which there is nuclear replication without plasmotomy (i.e. without division) and then two to many merozoites or daughter cells are produced simultaneously; a type of schizogony in which merozoites are formed; examples are found in many members of the Apicomplexa, such as *Eimeria* and *Plasmodium*.

**Merozoite:** product of merogony; usually an elongate organism that infects another host cell to undergo either merogony again or gamogony.

**Metacercaria (-iae):** infective stage of a fluke enclosed in a protective cyst that resists adverse environmental conditions. This stage develops from the cercaria and is infective for the definitive host.

**Metacestode:** immature tapeworm that develops from the hexacanth embryo (oncosphere) and grows in the intermediate host (mammal), but one not yet sexually mature.

**Microfilaria:** stage of filarial worm transmitted to the biting insect from the definitive host.

**Miracidium:** first developmental stage larva of a fluke; hatches from the egg and penetrates the snail intermediate host.

**Moulting (= ecdysis):** shedding of an external covering such as integument or exoskeleton; in arthropods and nematodes, shedding the external covering allows the parasite to expand in its new skin.

**Nymph:** preadult stage of an insect.

**Oncomiracidium:** free-swimming, ciliated larva of members of the Subclass Monogenea.

**Oncosphere:** six-hooked embryo that is contained in the egg membranes of members of the Class Cestoda. *See* Hexacanth.

**Oocyst:** stage in the life cycle of certain members of the Phylum Apicomplexa in which the zygote secretes a wall around itself; often highly resistant to environmental conditions.

**Operculum:** lid or cap-like structure at one or both ends of certain worm eggs (i.e. fluke); the larval parasite emerges from the egg at the operculum.

**Paratenic host:** host in which there is no development of the immature parasite; this host does not favour or hinder the parasite in the completion of its life cycle. The parasite may exist for longer periods here than in a transport host.

**Patent infection:** mature infection that is producing immature stages such as eggs or oocysts.

**Permanent parasites:** spend most of their life cycle in association with their hosts.

**Plasmotomy:** a type of asexual reproduction in which a protozoan cell divides into two or more multinucleate daughter cells.

**Plerocercoid:** larva or metacestode developing from a procercoid in the life cycle of tapeworms of the order Pseudophyllidea; this type of tapeworm larva is solid and has a rudimentary holdfast at the anterior end.

**Procercoid:** larva or metacestode that does not have a scolex similar to that of the adult tapeworm; commonly found in members of the tapeworm order Pseudophyllidea.

**Proglottid:** body segment of a tapeworm containing a complete set of reproductive organs.

# Glossary

Protoscolex (protoscolices): holdfast of tapeworms of the order Cyclophyllidea, which forms from a germinal epithelium in a coenurus or hydatid cyst.

Questing: process whereby ticks wait for a suitable host to pass them by before attaching to the host.

Redia: trematode stage in the snail intermediate host that develops from the sporocyst and becomes the cercaria.

Reportable disease: disease that, by law, must be reported to a health authority.

Reservoir host: infected definitive host serving as a source from which other animals or humans can become infected. The reservoir host never suffers from such association.

Rostellum: prominence on the anterior end of the scolex of certain tapeworms of the order Cyclophyllidea. Usually fitted with rows of hooks.

Schizogony: type of asexual reproduction in which there are multiple nuclear divisions and then plasmotomy takes place, giving rise to a large number of daughter cells; occurs often in members of the Phylum Apicomplexa; merogony and microgametogony are types of schizogony.

Scolex (scolices): holdfast or organ by which a tapeworm attaches to the intestine of its host.

Scutum: hard plate or shield on the dorsum behind the capitulum of hard ticks. Much more extensive in male than in female ticks.

Spicule (= copulatory spicule): an elongate, sclerotized structure of male nematodes used in holding open the vulva of the female during copulation and transfer of sperm.

Sporocysts: stage within oocysts that contains the sporozoites.

Sporogony: type of schizogony in which the product is the sporozoite.

Sporozoite: cellular infective stage in some members of the Phylum Apicomplexa. Evolves from excystation of oocysts and sporocysts.

Sylvatic: refers to a forest or a wooded area; used as an adjective to describe the location of a disease cycle in the wild.

Tachyzoite: fast-reproducing parasite stages within the host cell.

Temporary parasites: visit their hosts occasionally and at intermittent times for taking their meal (e.g. mosquitoes, bugs).

Transport host: host that is not needed for the parasite to complete any stage of its life cycle but is merely used to carry the non-developing parasite to the next host without further development (e.g. earthworm may ingest eggs or larvae and disseminate them as they pass through its gut).

Trophozoite: growing, feeding stage of a protozoan. In some species it is also called the vegetative stage.

Vector: agent of transmission. When the final or intermediate host that delivers the infectious agents to the animal or human is an arthropod it is defined as a vector (e.g. ticks act as a vector host for *Babesia* and mosquitoes act as a vector for malaria).

Vertical transmission: transmission of a parasite from one generation to the next through the egg or *in utero*.

Zoonosis (-es): diseases that are transmitted from animals to humans.

Zoonotic: an organism that causes a zoonosis.

# Host index

# Parasite index

# Parasite index

# General index

# General index

# General index

# General index